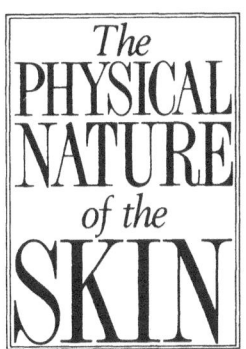

The
PHYSICAL
NATURE
of the
SKIN

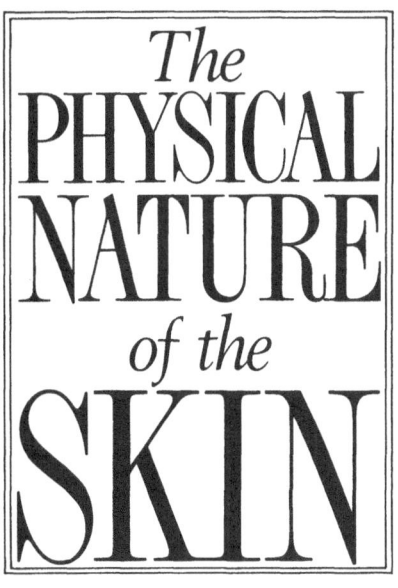

The
PHYSICAL
NATURE
of the
SKIN

Edited by

R.M.Marks S.P.Barton and C.Edwards

Department of Medicine (Dermatology)
University of Wales College of Medicine
Cardiff

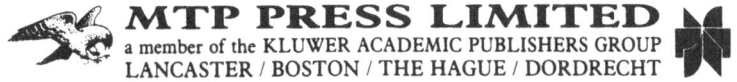

MTP PRESS LIMITED
a member of the KLUWER ACADEMIC PUBLISHERS GROUP
LANCASTER / BOSTON / THE HAGUE / DORDRECHT

Published in the UK and Europe by
MTP Press Limited
Falcon House
Lancaster, England

British Library Cataloguing in Publication Data

The Physical nature of the skin.
    1. Skin
    I. Marks, R.M.   II. Barton, S.P.
    III. Edwards, C.
    612'.79   QP88.5

Published in the USA by
MTP Press
A division of Kluwer Academic Publishers
101 Philip Drive
Norwell, MA 02061, USA

Library of Congress Cataloging-in-Publication Data

The Physical nature of the skin.

    Includes bibliographies and index.
    1. Skin. I. Marks, Ronald. II. Barton, S. P.
(Steven P.) III. Edwards, C. (Christopher)
[DNLM: 1. Skin--anatomy & histology. 2. Skin--
physiology. WR 100 P578]
QP88.5.P475 1987   612'.79   87-31126
ISBN-13: 978-94-010-7074-4   e-ISBN-13: 978-94-009-1291-5
DOI: 10.1007/978-94-009-1291-5

Contents

List of contributors

J C Barbenel
Bioengineering Unit
University of Strathclyde
Wolfson Centre
Glasgow G4 0NW

B W Barry
Pharmaceutical Technology
University of Bradford
Richmond Road
Bradford BD7 1DP

S P Barton
Dept of Medicine (Dermatology)
University of Wales College of
    Medicine
Heath Park
Cardiff CF4 4XN

D R Black
Dept of Medicine (Dermatology)
University of Wales College of
    Medicine
Heath Park
Cardiff CF4 4XN

S M Breathnach
Dept of Medicine (Dermatology)
Charing Cross and Westminster
    Medical School
Fulham Palace Road
London W6 4XN

A Compston
Dept of Medicine (Neurology)
University of Wales College of
    Medicine
Heath Park
Cardiff CF4 4XN

M F Corbett
St John's Hospital for Diseases
    of the Skin
Lisle St
Leicester Square
London WC2H 7BJ

B L Diffey
Regional Medical Physics Dept
Dryburn Hospital
Durham DH1 5TW

C Edwards
Dept of Medicine (Dermatology)
University of Wales College of
    Medicine
Heath Park
Cardiff CF4 4XN

A Y Finlay
Dept of Medicine (Dermatology)
University of Wales College of
    Medicine
Heath Park
Cardiff CF4 4XN

M I Foreman
Data Analysis and Research Ltd
The Bell Tower
New Lanark
Lanarkshire ML11 9DH

C M Lapière
Dept of Dermatology
Université de Liège
Hôpital de Bavière, Bd de la
    Constitution, 66
B-4020 Liège
Belgium

J C Lawrence
MRC Burns Research Group
Birmingham Accident Hospital
Bath Row
Birmingham B15 1NA

J-L Lévêque
Dept Biophysique
Laboratoire de Research de
    L'OREAL
1, Avenue Eugène Schueller
93600 - Aulnay-sous-Bois Cedex
France

R Marks
Dept of Medicine (Dermatology)
University of Wales College of
    Medicine
Heath Park
Cardiff CF4 4XN

B B Michniak-Mikolajczak
Pharmaceutical Technology
University of Bradford
Richmond Road
Bradford BD7 1DP

B V Nusgens
Laboratoire de Dermatologie
    Expérimentale
Université de Liège
Tour de Pathologie, 3ème étage
B-4000 Sart Tilman par Liège 1
Belgium

P A Payne
Dept of Instrumentation and
    Analytical Science
UMIST
PO Box 88
Manchester M60 1QD

C M Philpot
Dept of Medical Microbiology
University Hospital of Wales
Heath Park
Cardiff CF4 4XW

G E Pierard
Dept of Dermatology
Université de Liège
Hôpital de Bavière, Bd de la
    Constitution, 66
B-4020 Liège
Belgium

L Rasseneur
Dept Biophysique
Laboratoire de Research de
    L'OREAL
1, Avenue Eugène Schueller
93600 - Aulnay-sous-Bois Cedex
France

T J Ryan
Dept of Dermatology
Slade Hospital
Headington
Oxford OX3 7JH

J D Wilkinson
Dept of Dermatology
Wycombe General Hospital
High Wycombe
Bucks HP11 2TT

Foreword

R Marks

Skin is a fascinatingly complex structure. All of us whose lives revolve around its study are repeatedly surprised at the efficiency of its construction so carefully matched to its function. It is difficult to believe that further advances in our understanding of the nature of skin can be made without paying attention to its physical characteristics as well as by pursuing the more traditional biochemical approach to its study. There must also be benefits to skin biology from the incorporation of the new physical techniques and non-invasive methods of interrogating tissues. It is with these issues in mind that a symposium was held in Cardiff, on which this book is based. The contributors are all active researchers in one or another aspect of the subject and we hope that this has ensured both scholarship and the air of excitement so necessary to effective research.

We make no apology for this volume not including all possible physical studies of skin. For the most part the selection reflects our own interests and assessment as to relevance. Nonetheless, we believe that the volume does underline the physical basis for the maintenance of the skin's organization overall, both as a supporting connective tissue and a renewable protective layer. We also hope that it will show how much these interdependent parts interact with each other and their environment. As such the book should be of interest to all who have the care of skin at the centre of their professional lives.

Section I

ORGANIZATION AND DIMENSIONS OF THE SKIN

Chapter 1

Skin under the microscope: the organization, kinetics and dimensions of skin

R Marks

A histological tyranny has subverted dermatologists and skin biologists and impeded a better understanding of how the skin behaves either at rest or after challenge in some way. The conventional histological section represents a tiny part of the entire integuement seen in two dimensions and at one point in time. This inability to view anything other than a fragment of skin 'frozen in time' is not the only problem with the conventional histological section. What is seen down the microscope has been chemically assaulted by fixation, dehydration, wax impregnation and staining as well as having been physically battered by the sectioning technique. It seems unlikely that anything but the grossest changes will be evident. To gain insight into interrelationships within skin and to obtain information concerning skin function we need to use a variety of other techniques. It is my intention in this chapter to encourage readers to appreciate and even surmount the constraints implicit in the histological approach. There are constraints of space and time.

SPATIAL CONSTRAINTS

A major limitation to an understanding of the nature of normal or diseased organs by examining their histological structure is that with few exceptions, organs are not homogenous structures, and it is unlikely that the sample obtained will accurately represent the whole part of interest. This problem is compounded in the histological study of disease as it is uncommon for a disease process to affect an organ uniformly, regardless of whether infection, trauma, neoplasia or metabolic inadequacy is the cause. The problem is particularly pronounced with skin, as it is an amalgam of closely intertwined tissues. To illustrate the difficulties that arise because of undue emphasis on the histological approach, I will cite examples based at both ends of the dimensional spectrum.

It has always been of interest to me that nuclear fragments are hardly ever seen in the granular cell layer of the epidermis, despite the fact that all keratinocytes destined to become corneocytes lose their nuclei. Fragments are occasionally seen by electron microscopy, but hardly ever by light microscopy. Presumably this odd apparent absence of an event that we know must take place is due both to the short-lived nature of the event and the difficulties of identifying nuclear fragments in a flattened granular cell that also contains basophilic granules of keratohyalin.

Apoptosis is the process of programmed intratissue cell death[1]. It seems likely that this process plays some role in the population dynamics of the epidermis but because apoptotic bodies have been difficult to identify in the normal epidermis it has been difficult to believe that it is physiologically important. Perhaps this is analogous to the invisibility of nuclear fragments, and is the result of the relatively small size of apoptotic bodies and their relative infrequency.

Identification of the hyphal elements of dermatophyte fungus within the stratum corneum of a biopsy from a lesion of ringworm may be very difficult, even with special stains, because of the sparseness of the microorganism. It is universally recognized that there are more efficient methods of diagnosis of ringworm than by biopsy. Microscopic examination of scraped-off scale in KOH or of skin surface biopsy and PAS staining[2] are much more likely to yield positive results (Figure 1.1) Similar considerations apply to the identification of sparsely distributed structures more deeply embedded within the skin, and we need techniques analogous to skin surface biopsy to detect them.

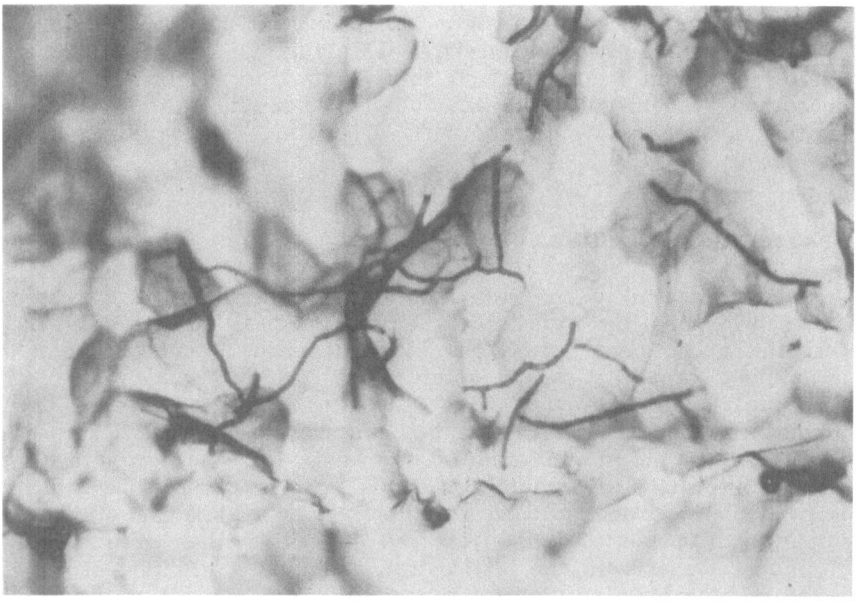

Figure 1.1 Skin surface biopsy from ringworm lesion stained with periodic acid Schiff reagent to show hyphal forms of ringworm. With this technique it is quite easy to see the infecting microorganisms within the stratum corneum

We can improve our chances of detecting a rare event or a sparsely distributed structure in a number of ways. The simplest is to increase the number of samples examined by taking 'step sections' in which the tissue is examined by looking at sections mounted at regular intervals throughout the sample or by serially sectioning the sample in which adjacent sections are mounted and inspected. It should be appreciated that with the average 5 μm thick histological section and not taking into account shrinkage due to processing, trimming and wastage, there will be some 200 sections per millimetre length of tissue. Clearly, it is only possible to examine samples, and not every last cell of these.

There is a better chance of detecting the required phenomenon if it is known in which part of the skin it is likely to reside and it is possible to somehow 'concentrate' this particular part. The skin surface biopsy technique[3,4] will permit the stratum corneum to be studied at any depth. It is also possible to horizontally section the skin in an attempt at sampling the epidermis or the dermis at a particular level. Unfortunately, because of the tendency of skin samples to 'curl at the edges' on account of the pull of the dermal elements after releasing in vivo tensions (Figure 1.2), horizontal sections inevitably contain tissues from a variety of depths (Figure 1.3).

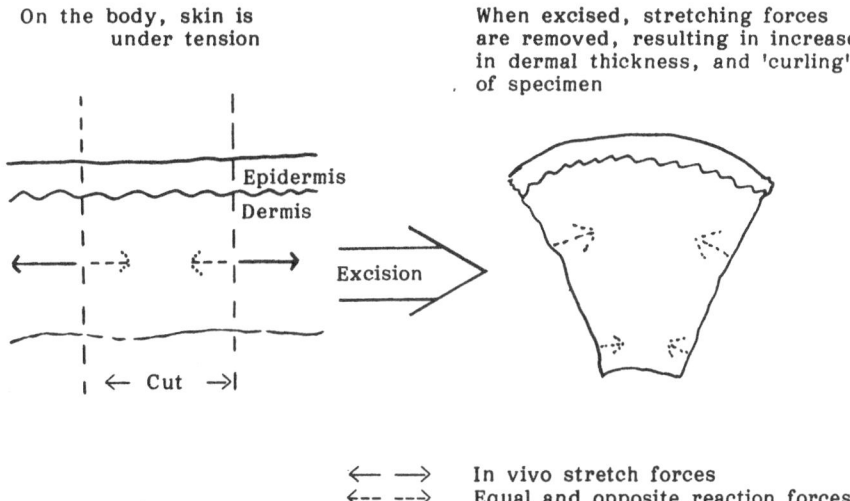

Figure 1.2 On excision, in vivo tension is released, resulting in dermal contraction which 'curls' the specimen

Alternatively it may be possible to disaggregate the tissue and either concentrate the cell type of interest or culture it. This approach is certainly feasible for keratinocytes and fibroblasts. Although not yet routine, it is also possible to investigate melanocytes[5], apocrine cells[6] and capillary endothelial cells[7] using cultural methods. The disadvantage of this approach is our uncertainty that events seen in vitro entirely mimic the situation in vivo. Furthermore, there are some cell types, such as Langerhans cells, that have steadfastly resisted cultural methods. Another way of inspecting the skin in the horizontal dimension is to split the epidermis from the dermis to study the bottom of the former or the top of the latter (Figure 1.4) but there are limited applications for this.

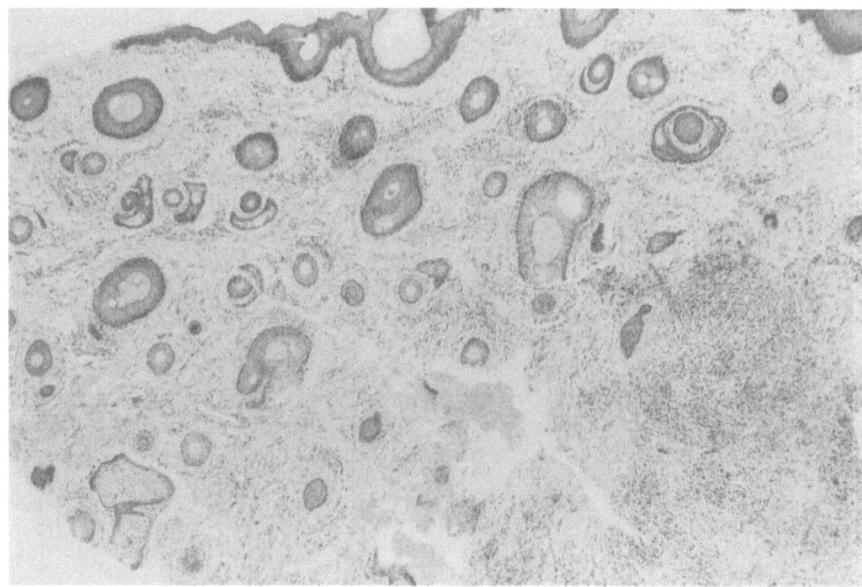

Figure 1.3 Horizontal section from skin of the face. Skin from several layers, including epidermis, has been included because the edges of the specimen have curled over

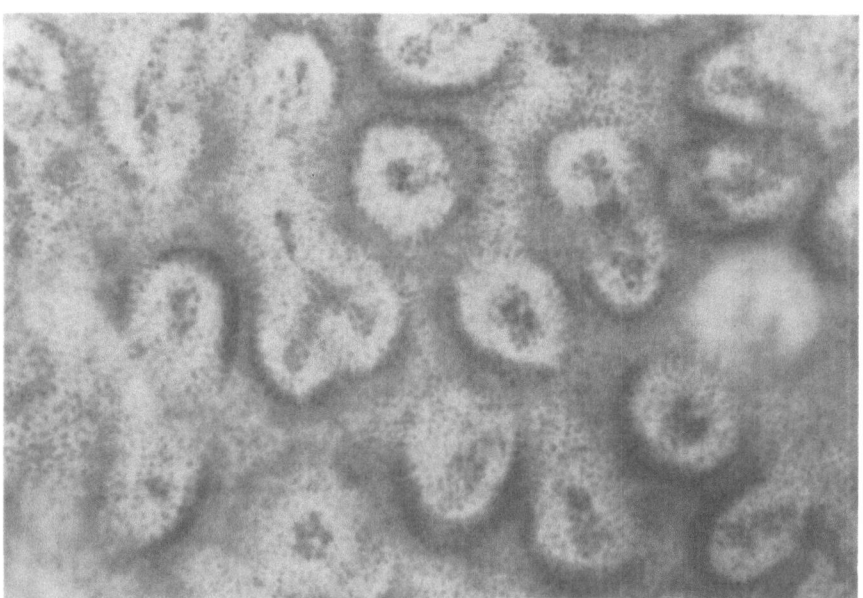

Figure 1.4 Photomicrograph of epidermis after dermal-epidermal split, using 0.05% trypsin. Many rounded areas where the dermis projects into the epidermis can be seen

By examining the tissue using ultrastructural methods we can ensure that we have not missed structures because they are less than a micron in size. In addition, there is an improved chance of visualizing delicate membranes that are destroyed by histological processing but preserved by the more gentle fixatives used in electron microscopy.

At the other end of the scale of dimensions, it is impossible to know from a biopsy what proportion of the body surface is affected by a disease process. It is a bit like studying the arrangement of the planets with a microscope rather than a telescope. If a lesion on the arm is biopsied, is this necessarily representative of a lesion on the abdomen or on the scalp? How can we know that lesions are orientated along the long axis of a limb, in the distribution of the dorsal nerve roots or restricted to extensor aspects of the body, merely by examining a histological section? Humanitarian and

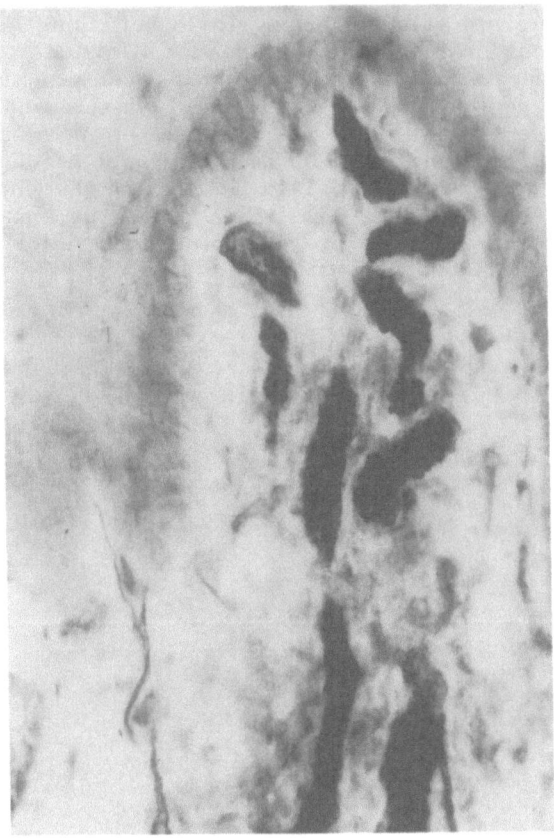

Figure 1.5 Photomicrograph of 20 μm thick section which has been reacted for adenosine triphosphatase activity. This high power view of a dermal papilla shows the pattern of the papillary capillary because of the thickness of the section

7

practical considerations aside, it is almost impossible to obtain an accurate view of the totality of involvement of the skin organ in a disease process by taking multiple biopsies.

There is one other major disadvantage of the routine histological technique and that is, regardless of any confusion induced by the inherent sampling error, it is very difficult to obtain information concerning the arrangement of tissues from a two-dimensional section. Unless a picture is built up from serial sections we can only guess at the significance of the shape of tissues, and will have little idea as to tissue interrelationships. For example, it is almost impossible to obtain any detailed picture of the surface patterning of the stratum corneum using conventional histological techniques. The same is true of the arrangement of the dermo-epidermal junction. For these last two purposes it is necessary to examine the appropriate part of the skin in the horizontal dimension, using the skin surface biopsy or skin replica technique in the one case and dermo-epidermal separation in the other. These are special examples in which there are suitable techniques to surmount the difficulties. Other questions involving the arrangement of structures in a three-dimensional aspect are less easily tackled. 'Thick sections' of up to 20 μm thick can be used to stain blood vessels and nerves and sometimes other structures to get some idea of their disposition in a small segment of skin (Figure 1.5). Horizontal sections parallel to the skin surface may be used to look at the distribution of some elements in this dimension where this cannot be answered by the routine preparation. It was quite helpful, for example, in characterizing the role of follicular structures in rosacea[8] (Figure 1.6).

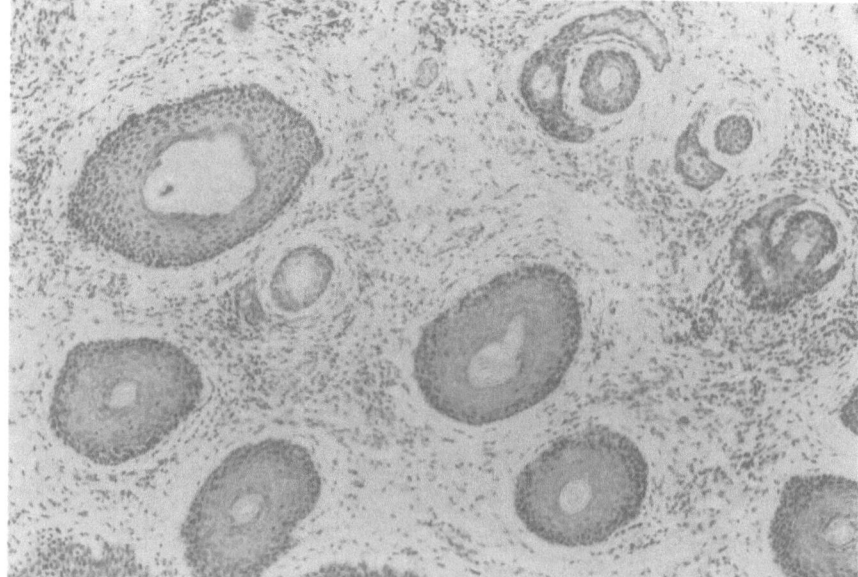

Figure 1.6 Horizontal section of facial skin in rosacea. The section shows many follicular elements. There was no curling in the case of this specimen (see Figure 1.3)

KINETIC CONSTRAINTS

The real deceit of the histological section is its static nature. Skin is anything but static. It has always astonished me that it succeeds in performing its manifold functions on the hoof, so to speak. The stratum corneum protects while desquamating, the dermis binds, conforms and protects while metabolizing and renewing, and the whole organ heals when injured, and so on. Morphological techniques are not often able to, or indeed designed to, inform on function, but there are ways of learning something of the way skin behaves from special preparative methods. For example, presentation of a radioactively labelled specific precursor of DNA (tritiated thymidine) either in vitro or by intracutaneous injection in vivo to skin and subsequent autoradiographic processing[9] will label all the cells undergoing DNA synthesis and about to divide (Figure 1.7).

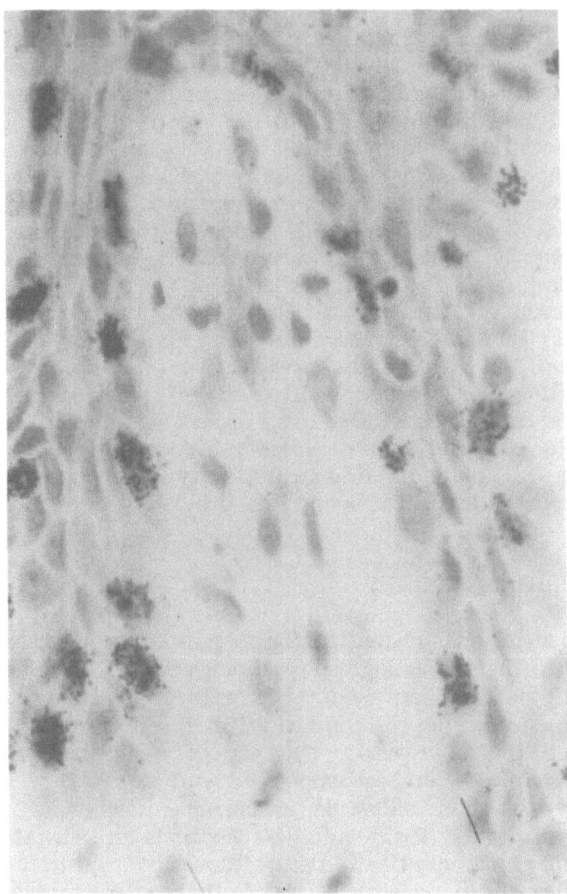

Figure 1.7 Autoradiograph to show many autoradiographically labelled cells after injection of tritiated thymidine in vivo in a lesion of lichenified eczema. Many cells can be seen in the basal layer of the epidermis over which are silver grains, indicating that the cell has incorporated the isotopically labelled thymidine and is in the process of DNA synthesis

Subsequent assessment of the number of labelled epidermal cells in the basal and suprabasal layer as a proportion of the total number of cells in the basal layer (labelling index) allows some estimate of the proliferative status of the epidermis - albeit somewhat crudely.

Other so-called 'stathmokinetic' methods allow estimation of the number of cells entering mitosis per hour. Colcemid (a colchicine alkaloid) or vincristine (a vinca - periwinkle - alkaloid) stops cells in the metaphase stage of mitosis. Tissue is presented with one of these agents 4 hours previously and the number of basal cells arrested is counted and expressed as a proportion of the whole basal layer, allowing an estimate of the proportion of cells entering mitosis per hour.

More sophisticated methods now permit cells in the mitotic cycle to be labelled by an immunocytochemical technique. A monoclonal antibody known as Ki67 labels the dividing cells, and using a peroxidase system it is relatively easy to detect and count them microscopically. Disaggregation of epidermal tissue, either fixed or unfixed, allows the nuclear DNA to be stoichiometrically labelled with propidium iodide and fluoresce according to the amount of DNA present. By running the labelled cell dispersion through a fluorescence activated cell sorting (FACS) device, it is possible to determine the number of cells in DNA synthesis.

Enzyme cytochemical and immunocytochemical methods allow identification, localization and indeed quantification of enzyme activities and the presence of immunogenic substances in the tissue. Clearly it is possible to learn something of the function of tissue and the pathodynamics of disease from these types of 'static' preparations for the microscope. But no matter the degree of sophistication and care in the preparative technique, the constraints of the histological method still exist - the microscope section represents a tiny piece of the total organ being examined. It is seen in two dimensions and after a variety of damaging chemical assaults. In my view, histological information may well be important but it must always be interpreted alongside other types of data.

THE DIMENSIONS OF SKIN

Merely inspecting tissue and making qualitative judgements has been the stuff of all morphological pathology until recently. But now much more information can be extracted using morphometric (histometric) techniques. Surprisingly, it is possible to assess the thickness of the epidermis, the size of epidermal cells, stratum corneum thickness and corneocyte surface area using simple microscope projection side-arm measurement methods[10]. Of course the use of automated image analysis methods speeds things up, but the principles are identical. Using these conceptually fairly simple methods it has been possible to show that epidermal cells enlarge in acromegaly[11] and decrease in size after treatment with corticosteroids[12] - facts that do not seem to have been suspected by mere inspection of sections. We have also shown that epidermal cells decrease in size with age[10]. By employing the parameter of mean keratinocyte height (MKh) it was found that cells decreased from a mean value of approximately 12.5 μm MKh at the age of 20 to about 7.5 μm at the age of 85. Such measurements are of value in research - whether they will also be of value in routine care is another issue. It is likely that some such measurement technique will be of clinical value at some point in the future.

The above are very simple measurement techniques. As you may have guessed, there are also much more sophisticated methods that enable accurate estimates to be made of the volume (or other dimensions) of any structure. These techniques rely on random sampling and the use of grids, enabling projections to be made in three dimensions. These stereological methods are outlined in more detail in the next chapter in discussion of measurement at the ultrastructural level but they can certainly be employed using ordinary 'paraffin' sections as well - as, for example, in the measurement of the size of the components of the pilosebaceous apparatus in the condition senile sebaceous gland hyperplasia[13].

CONCLUSION

I would not wish the reader to believe that there is little to be learnt from histological sections. The opposite is the case. An enormous amount of information can be gleaned - with two provisos. The first of these is that the very real limitations must be recognized. If one takes these into account and uses any other information that is required, it will be possible to make reasonable interpretations. The other is that it should be appreciated that a variety of other methods exist to expand, qualify and quantify the information from what is after all only a tiny bit of distorted tissue, and these should be used when appropriate.

REFERENCES

1. Kerr, J.F.R., Wyllie, A.H. and Currie, A.R. (1972). Apoptosis: a basic biological phenomenon with wide ranging implications in tissue kinetics. Br. J. Cancer, **26**, 329-33
2. Marks, R. and Dawber, R.P.R. (1972). In situ microbiology of the stratum corneum. Arch. Dermatol., **105**, 216-21
3. Marks, R. and Dawber, R.P.R. (1971). Skin surface biopsy: an improved technique for the examination of the horny layer. Br. J. Dermatol., **84**, 117-23
4. Marks, R. (1972). Histochemical applications of skin surface biopsy. Br. J. Dermatol., **86**, 20-6
5. Eisinger, M. and Marko, O. (1982). Selective proliferation of normal human melanocytes in vitro in the presence of phorbol ester and cholera toxin. Proc. Natl. Acad. Sci. USA, 1979. pp 2018-22
6. Harrison, B.J., Jones, D.L. and Hughes, L.E. (1987). Growth of apocrine cells in tissue culture. Abstract of paper presented at 17th Annual Meeting of European Society for Dermatological Research, Amsterdam, March-April
7. Davison, P.M., Bensch, K. and Karasek, M.A. (1980). Isolation and growth of endothelial cells from the microvessels of the newborn human foreskin in cell culture. J. Invest. Dermatol., **75**, 316-21
8. Marks, R. and Harcourt-Webster, J.N. (1969). Histopathology of rosacea. Arch. Dermatol., **100**, 683-92
9. Shahrad, P. and Marks, R. (1976). Hair follicle kinetics in psoriasis. Br. J. Dermatol., **94**, 7-12

10. Marks, R. (1981). Measurement of biological ageing in human epidermis. Br. J. Dermatol., **104**, 627-33
11. Holt, P.J.A. and Marks, R. (1976). Epidermal architecture, growth and metabolism in acromegaly. Br. Med. J., **1**, 496-7
12. Delfarno, C., Holt, P.J.A. and Marks, R. (1978). Corticosteroid effect on epidermal cell size. Br. J. Dermatol., **98**, 619-23
13. Kumar, P., Barton, S.P. and Marks, R. (1987). Tissue measurements in senile sebaceous gland hyperplasia. Br. J. Dermatol., (in press)

Chapter 2

Epidermal dimensions at the ultrastructural level

S P Barton

INTRODUCTION

In most structural studies the tissue under examination is killed by fixation. This effectively reduces the opportunity to examine changes in time and we are left with three spatial dimensions. It is important to appreciate that in most instances the three-dimensional configuration of a tissue is seen as a two-dimensional section. When attempting to quantify dimensions this two-dimensional representation of structure plays an important role in influencing the values derived and affecting the sample size required, which is enormous in the case of ultrastructural observations. To understand the importance of dimensions, it is necessary to study the means of achieving such quantities and the potential errors in their interpretation. To examine one ultrathin section at 10 000 x magnification and extrapolate this sole observation to the whole tissue is akin to examining one blue wall in one room of a multi-storey block and concluding that the whole building is probably blue.

In this contribution I shall demonstrate some of the options open to anyone interested in pursuing a quantitative study of skin dimensions at the ultrastructural level. It is not the purpose of this chapter to be a full exposition of the art of measurement, since this is available elsewhere[1-3]. Whilst specific examples will be given here, the reader can refer to several other quantitative studies of epidermis which have appeared in the literature[4-7].

RESOLUTION AND CALIBRATION

Measurement is simple given the appropriate image. Whichever way the image is subsequently treated, it can be considered to be a matrix. The elements of this matrix may be silver grains on a photographic emulsion, squares of a graph paper, intersecting wires on a digitizer tablet or the picture elements (pixels) of a video camera. Each element represents the unit of measurement, prior to calibration, and this must be borne in mind when quantifying an image so that the real limit of resolution is known. Derivation of dimensions can then be seen in terms of these units as shown in Figure 2.1.

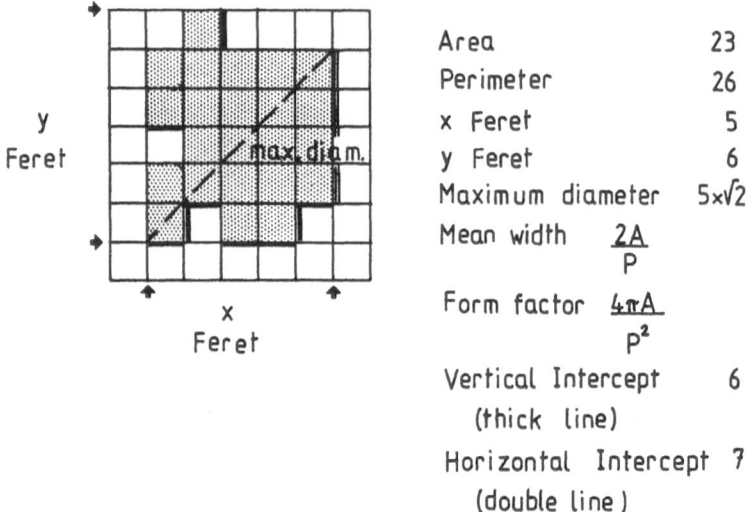

Area	23
Perimeter	26
x Feret	5
y Feret	6
Maximum diameter	5×√2

Mean width $\dfrac{2A}{P}$

Form factor $\dfrac{4\pi A}{P^2}$

Vertical Intercept (thick line)	6
Horizontal Intercept (double line)	7

Figure 2.1 The basic elements of measurement, represented as boxes, and the dimensions derived from a feature (shaded) defined in terms of these elements. Diagonal dotted lines = maximum diameter; solid horizontal lines = vertical intercept; double vertical lines = horizontal intercept. Arrows indicate extremes of feature in the x and y dimension (Feret diameters)

This figure also shows that magnification and resolution are not simply related. Figure 2.1 may be a magnified view of a TV screen but has no more resolution than the original image. Resolution is not a biological phenomenon, but a result of the process of generating the image. The classical analogy is the length of a coastline measured from maps of different scales[8]. The smaller the scale of the map, the larger the estimate of the coastline length. Similarly, tracing the length of cell membrane on a micrograph at 6000 x magnification would give different absolute dimensions than tracing the same length of cell membrane at twice this magnification. It is sufficient to alert you to this problem rather than answer the question, 'Which of these values represents the "truth"?', since this is dealt with more fully elsewhere; the interested reader is directed to Mandebrot's treatise on this problem[9].

This brings us to a subject which light microscopists treat far less seriously than any self-respecting electron microscopist - calibration. Routine operation of any modern electron microscope is as easy as a light microscope, but the conditions of lens current, filament current, aperture size and kV vary in a way that can affect the final magnification. Calibration is therefore essential for any study of tissue dimension.

Table 2.1 (Some) Epidermal dimensions at the ultrastructural level

Organelle	Dimension	Value(μm)
Nucleus	mean Feret	4.60
Nucleolus	mean Feret	1.22
Nuclear pore	maximum diameter	0.04
Tonofilament	maximum length	1.36
Mitochondrion	mean Feret	0.34
Golgi	maximum diameter	0.25
Endoplasmic reticulum	maximum diameter	0.49
Melanosome	mean Feret	0.24
Desmosome	length	0.26
Hemi-desmosome	length	0.19

Assuming that this has been duly considered, a table of measurements such as those in Table 2.1 could be easily generated from a series of randomly selected micrographs of the epidermis. Whilst all of the organelles are represented, the validity of the dimensions is dependent upon the resolution of the measurement. At the magnification chosen for these measurements, the Feret diameter of the nucleus will be more reliable than the Feret diameter of the nuclear pore, since the latter is close to the resolution of the digitizer tablet used. Another consequence of approaching the limit of resolution is that a limited number of values are possible for each profile. The mean and standard deviation derived would probably suggest a reasonably reproducible measurement.

SAMPLING AND REPRESENTATIVITY

Sectioning is a sampling procedure and apart from any compression artefacts, this itself may also influence the values derived. Since sections have a finite thickness, the magnitude of this in comparison to the dimension measured must be taken into account. Thus the sampling of nuclear pores in the measurements shown will be complete because their dimensions are less than the thickness of the section. Nuclei, being of far greater dimensions than ultrathin sections, will require more exhaustive sampling to obtain a full picture of variability in nuclear Feret diameter. The related phenomenon, known as Holmes effect[10], should also be considered. Simply stated, this shows that a particle will have different 'real' dimensions on either side of the section. This again relates to the finite thickness of the section in comparison to the dimension of the particle to be measured. For a more extensive description of the influence of sectioning upon dimensions, the reader should consult Aherne and Dunhill[1], Weibel[2] or Williams[3].

With the summary statistics from the above measurements, the dimensions could then be used to comment upon the size distribution or even the shape of particular organelles. The dimensions outlined in Figure 2.1 are but a few of the more commonly used descriptors of size. The form factor given is an indication of the roundness (i.e. a circle will have a form factor of 1) but a particular organelle may well command its own form factor.

Having briefly referred to the random sampling used to obtain the dimensions in Figure 2.1, it should now be clear that here is yet another consideration. For if these measurements were drawn randomly from a sufficient number of sections, then they would represent a mean value for the epidermis as a whole. There are various ways of ensuring that the number of measurements taken is in fact representative of the whole. The simplest, that described by Chalkey[11], is performed by calculating the cumulative standard error for each subsample (e.g. micrograph) and expressing it as a percentage of the mean. A plot of this against the number of subsamples will graphically show when additional measurements have no further effect on the magnitude of the quantity derived. It has the added bonus of showing the expected standard error of the measurement. The method of selecting the particular regions of the tissue to be subsampled is a related problem. Random sampling or systematic selection both have their value and readers are once again referred to general texts on measurement for a full analysis of this[1-3].

It has already been stated that sectioning itself is a sampling procedure and yet few dermatologists would consider looking at random sections of the epidermis. The stratified nature of the epidermis encourages us to observe it in the plane of a vertical section and the heterogeneity that this fact implies can and should be studied. In a study of desmosomes in the epidermis of normal and ichthyotic individuals, we separated the observations into three classes - those from the basal region, the spinous and granular layer, and the stratum corneum. In this way we hoped to examine whether there was a change in the distribution of these structures during differentiation. Figure 2.2 shows the numbers and lengths of desmosomes in normal epidermis and how these properties are distributed in the different strata. Whilst there is an obvious difference in the number per field, there is little difference in the size.

INTERPRETATION

Now the question arises - what does this difference in numbers mean? Interpretation is important, for if the result is taken at face value an essential feature of the process of differentiation may be overlooked. The amount of membrane available for desmosomes may also change in the same manner. The same argument can be applied to other measurements. The appropriate quality must be chosen when making any quantitative assessment of tissue. With many computer-assisted devices a number of parameters can be derived simultaneously (see Figure 2.1). In these cases it is a simple process to collect as many parameters from each image as it is

16

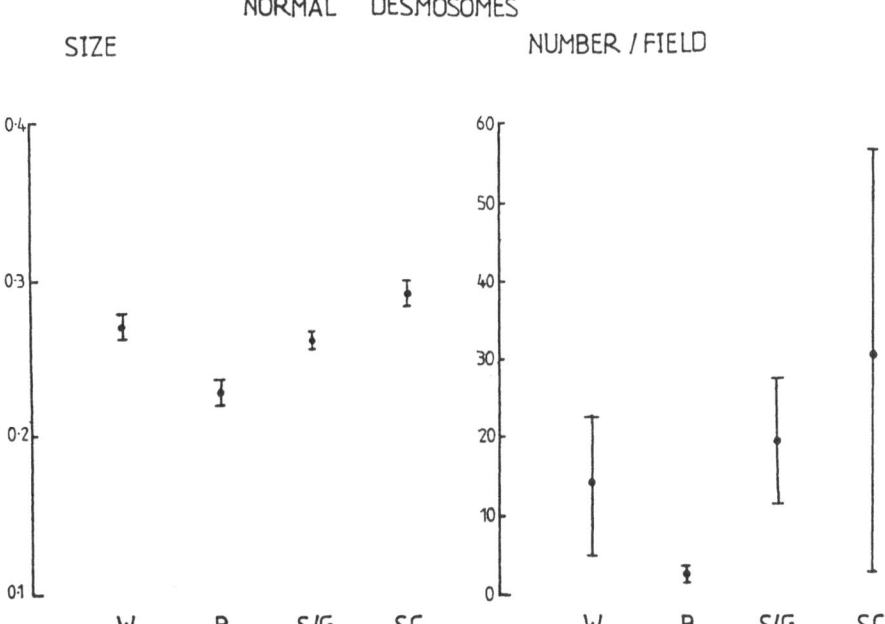

Figure 2.2 Size and number of desmosomes within the different compartments of the epidermis showing how the stratification affects the value. W = whole epidermis; B = basal layer; S/G = spinous/granular layer; SC = stratum corneum

possible to store. However, one can still be left puzzling what the significance of mitochondrial Feret diameters means biologically. Does a cell with few mitochondria of large Feret diameter have any advantage over one with many small organelles?

Posing a similar question in the case of desmosomes, is the length or size the most important parameter to assess? It has been suggested that the proportion of the membrane occupied by desmosome is a more relevant measure of cell to cell attachment[12] than size distribution or number alone. This could be done planimetrically if the membrane could be viewed en face but this is impossible in whole biopsies. Using the elegant technique of stereology, measurements of surface area of desmosome and membrane can easily be made from sections. Stereological methods are explained at length elsewhere[1-3] but it may be useful to describe the logic of their use here.

A section represents a two-dimensional sample of a three-dimensional object (see Figure 2.3). If the object is contained within a reference space, then on average, the area fraction of the object in the reference space section is equal to the relative volume of that object in that space. A one-dimensional section of this two-dimensional profile will similarly measure the relative area. A nought-dimensional section (points) will hence measure the relative

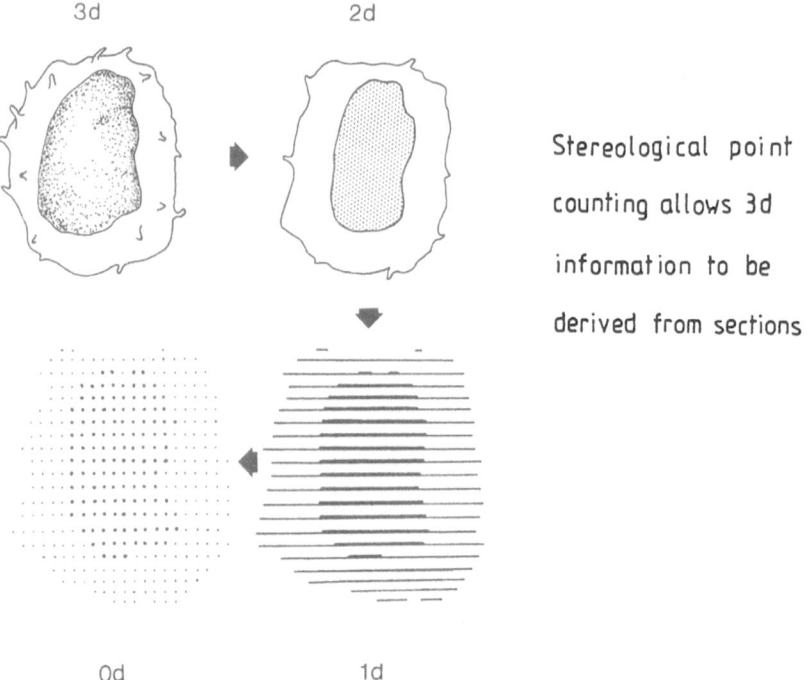

Figure 2.3 A cell sectioned into its component dimensions showing how 0-dimensional points can represent volume estimations (3-dimensions)

length of the line. So, by superimposing a lattice of points on an adequate number of micrographs, and counting those contained within certain objects, we can gain an estimate of the relative volume taken up by those objects in a reference volume. The reader is referred to other texts for the constraints and factors influencing choice of reference volume, point lattice spacing, and numbers of micrographs required[1-3].

For the purposes of estimating the relative surface area occupied by desmosomes on the keratinocyte membrane the logic has to be extended one stage further. Just as a lattice of points will sample the relative volume of organelles, so a lattice of 'needles' will effectively sample the surface area of membrane and associated structures. This is achieved by counting the number of intersections of the test lines with the keratinocyte membrane. This will be an estimate of membrane surface area and the number of times the lines cut a desmosome profile will therefore be a measure of the proportion of the keratinocyte membrane occupied by desmosome. To contend with the anisotropy of the epidermis we have used the curvilinear sampling method of Merz[13]. This allows the stratum corneum to be sampled without orientation influencing the result.

18

The amount of membrane per unit volume of epidermis can thus be shown to be responsible for the increased numbers of desmosomes observed in our sample of ichthyotics. Figure 2.4 shows this, there being more keratinocyte membrane in the ichthyotics we have observed so far. When desmosomes are expressed as a fraction of the membrane surface area, the comparison between ichthyotics and normals is much closer (Figure 2.5).

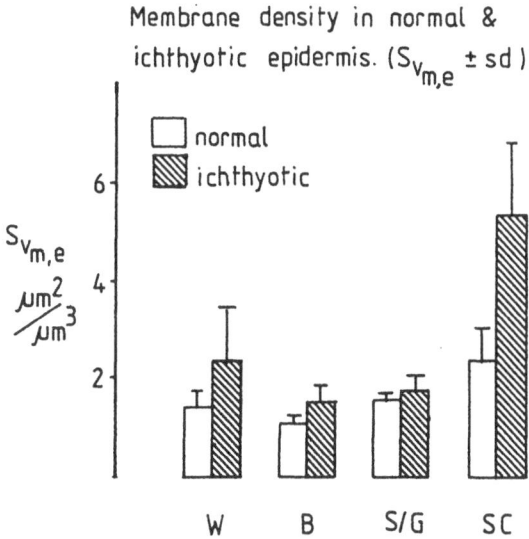

Figure 2.4 Stereological intersect counting to derive the amount of membrane per unit volume of epidermal tissue. Ichthyotic specimens appear to have more membrane per unit volume. W = whole epidermis; B = basal layer; S/G = spinous/granular layer; SC = stratum corneum

The method can be expanded to include the ratio of membrane (or other) surface area to the volume. This may be necessary when quantifying mitochondria or lamellar bodies, where function may be related to the surface:volume ratio. Again this returns to the biological consequences of the parameters measured. The measurements in Table 2.1 are just a few of those possible in the epidermis, but are they of biological significance?

Nuclear shape may be better estimated at the ultrastructural level because of the increased resolution. A change in nuclear shape or a departure from normal has been suggested as an indication of neoplastic change[14]. Tidman and Eady have tirelessly measured the hemi-desmosome number and length as well as the distribution of dermal anchoring fibrils in normal individuals and various epidermolytic disorders[15]. Their work also underlined the variability brought about by sampling different body sites. Unfortunately, their results did not permit them to offer any strong guidance on

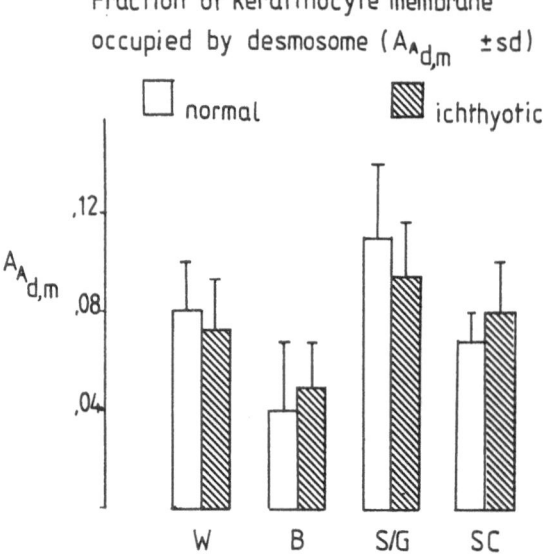

Fraction of keratinocyte membrane
occupied by desmosome $(A_{A_{d,m}} \pm sd)$

☐ normal   ▨ ichthyotic

Figure 2.5 The fraction of keratinocyte membrane occupied by desmosomes, estimated by stereological intersect counting. Little difference can be seen between normal and ichthyotic specimens. W = whole epidermis; B = basal layer; S/G = spinous/granular layer; SC = stratum corneum

the diagnostic use of the frequency of these structures in the epidermolysis bullosa disorders. At the other end of the epidermis, there has been a great deal of interest in the contribution of intercorneocyte space in percutaneous penetration. Following ultrastructural observation of a 'larger space', it has even been suggested that the reservoir capacity of the stratum corneum lies within this space[16]. Quantitative analysis is now required to substantiate this hypothesis. Difficulties in maintaining the stratum corneum structure in an 'in vivo' state during tissue preparation for electron microscopy have been thought to mitigate against this work being done. Whilst there may be a certain amount of truth in this, there is always room for comparative studies to point the way. I have deliberately left the question of fixation and preparative artefact to the end. As in all serious electron microscopy, reproducible artefact is what must be aimed for in dimensional studies at the ultrastructural level. Lindberg et al.[17,18] carefully showed the effect of fixation upon the intercellular volume of the epidermis before carrying out their quantitative studies on the effects of occlusion on the epidermis.

20

CONCLUSION

The foregoing examples are but a few of the possible epidermal systems that could be investigated in a quantitative manner. As advances in related fields such as immunocytochemistry and ultramicrotomy of frozen tissues are made, these possibilities increase. Further automation of the process of measuring by image analysers also removes the element of labour intensiveness that deters many from using quantitative methods of study. It is hoped that this contribution has at least caused some readers to accept that the quantitative approach has something to offer in spite of its apparent tedium in execution, and since more epidermal cell processes are beginning to be understood at a finer level it would be gratifying to see the structural consequences of these being assessed quantitatively in the future.

REFERENCES

1. Aherne, W.A. and Dunhill, M.S. (1982). Morphometry. (London: Edward Arnold)
2. Weibel, E.R. (1979). Stereological Methods. Vol. 1. Practical methods for biological morphometry. (New York: Academic Press)
3. Williams, M.A. (1977). Quantitative methods in biology. In Glauert, A.M. (ed.) Practical Methods in Electron Microscopy. Vol. 6. (Amsterdam: North Holland Publishing Co.)
4. Waterhouse, J.P. and Squier, C.A. (1969). Measurement of organelle size in relation to their shape: a refinement applied to the epidermal melanosome and basal lamella. J. Microscopy, 89, (2), 195
5. Klein-Szanto, A.J.P., Andersen, L. and Schroeder, H.E. (1976). Epithelial differentiation patterns in buccal mucosa affected by lichen planus. Virchows Arch. B Cell Pathol., 22, 245
6. Klein-Szanto, A.J.P. (1977). Stereologic baseline data of normal human epidermis. J. Investigative Dermatol., 68, (2), 73
7. Klein-Szanto, A.J.P. (1977). Clear and dark basal keratinocytes in human epidermis - a stereological study. J. Cutaneous Pathol., 4, 275
8. Mandelbrot, B.B. (1967). How long is the coast of Britain? Statistical self similarity and fractal dimension. Science, 155, 636
9. Mandelbrot, B.B. (1977). Fractals: Form, Chance, and Dimension. (San Francisco: Freeman and Co.)
10. Holmes, A.H. (1921). Petrographic Methods and Calculations. (London: Murby)
11. Chalkey, H.W. (1943). Method for quantitative morphologic analysis of tissue. J. Natl. Cancer Inst. 4, 47
12. White, F.H., Mayhew, T.M. and Gohari, K. (1982). Stereological methods for quantifying cell surface specialisations in epithelia, including a concept for counting desmosomes and hemi-desmosomes. Br. J. Dermatol., 107, 401
13. Merz, W.A. (1986). Streckenmessung an gerichtenen strukturen im Mikroskop und ihre Andwendung zur Bestimmung von Oberflachen-Volumen-relationen im Knochengewbe. Mikroskopie, 22, 132
14. Lessana-Leibowitch, M., Prado, A., Palangie, A., Lamy, F. and Flandrin, G. (1984). The diagnosis of cutaneous T-cell lymphomas by morphometric evaluation of the cellular infiltrate using semi-thin sections. Br. J. Dermatol., 110, 511
15. Tidman, M.J. and Eady, R.A.J. (1985). Evaluation of anchoring fibrils and other components of the dermal-epidermal junction in dystrophic epidermolysis bullosa by a quantitative ultrastructural technique. J. Invest. Dermatol. 84 (5), 374
16. Dupuis, D., Rougier, A., Roguet, R. and Lotte, C. (1986). The measurement of stratum corneum reservoir: simple method to predict the influence on in vivo percutaneous absorption. Br. J. Dermatol., 115 (2), 233
17. Lindberg, M. (1982). Variation in epidermal structure as a function of different fixation methods. A stereological and morphological study. Ph.D dissertation, Dept. of Medical Biophysics, Karolinska Institute, Stockholm, Sweden
18. Lindberg, M., Johannesson, A. and Forslind, B. (1982). The effect of occlusive treatment on human skin: an electron microscopic study on epidermal morphology as affected by occlusion and dansyl chloride. Dermato-Venerol. (Stockh.), 62, 1

Chapter 3

Surface contour: variability, significance and measurement

S P Barton and D R Black

INTRODUCTION

The surface of the skin is not only the part which we all see, but the barrier between ourselves and the environment. Subtle changes in this layer are therefore important from a pathological, physiological and cosmetic point of view. The organization of the stratum corneum is discussed elsewhere in this book, but here we will consider the methods available for the measurement of its free surface and what the measurements imply. In doing so it is important to understand the factors which contribute to the profile of the skin. Three orders of variation exist which may be thought of as three wavelengths. The longest of these is associated with the major skin furrows and 'wrinkles'. Superimposed upon this are smaller frequency variations due to local arrangement of the corneocytes. At the submicroscopic level there are also variations in the surface of the corneocytes themselves. However, there are other factors which do not affect the actual contour but influence an observer's impression of 'roughness' or 'scaliness'. These include skin colour, skin lipid composition and distribution, etc. and will not be dealt with here save to mention their contribution to the subjective analysis of skin contour.

The most obvious manifestations of skin contour changes can be seen in many of the scaling disorders of keratinization. However, this is not the only reason that surface contour measurements are required. The deep wrinkling observed in sun-exposed or aged skin can also be measured and this in itself may be related to, and therefore a measure of, skin elasticity. Hydration of the stratum corneum can have a marked effect upon the surface contour and analysis of this physical property can be used to assess hydration. In this way the change in surface contour occurring during therapy of the scaling disorders can be achieved using methods outlined below, as can the emollient effects of preparations used on normal but 'dry' skin.

In addition to the changes caused by pathology or treatment mentioned above, there are site- and age-specific variations which may be biologically interesting in themselves but also must be taken into account in any study of surface contour. The orientation of the major skin features is also an interesting phenomenon and this anisotropy can influence a measured quantity in skin contour analysis.

MEASUREMENT

Having commented upon the variability in skin contour and suggested some of the physical properties that this reflects, we must now consider the means by which the contour can be measured. However, it may be worthwhile to first look at the different surface characteristics which go to make up the whole 'surface contour'. In all the cases mentioned above a different component of the surface contour may be altered or changing, and it is therefore necessary to choose the appropriate parameter. Thus in wrinkled skin it may be that the extreme rather than the average depth of major features must be measured, whereas in 'dry' skin the frequency and amplitude of the surface between the major features may be more important. As in all science it is the relevance of the question asked which dictates the relevance of the answer. This leads us to a second consideration of the technique to be used - its resolution. The different 'wavelengths' of the contour vary by orders of magnitude, and so the resolution of the technique used has to be capable of detecting changes in the chosen parameter. The methods of assessing surface contour can be broadly categorized under three headings - subjective, mechanical and optical.

Subjective methods

The subjective methods are the most often used clinical tool incorporating the senses of sight and touch. Whilst they are purely subjective, attempts have been made to generate numbers and hence statistical analyses from such observations. Grading systems and visual analogue scales (VAS) are examples of this. Grading systems are of limited use but non-parametric statistics may be used to analyse such data[1]. The VAS method entails drawing a mark on a line of specified length (usually 100 mm) proportional to the observer's estimation of the quality being measured. The distance (in mm) from the origin of the line represents the quantification of this quality. Since this is a continuous scale it is apt to use conventional statistical methods. However, there are other difficulties with this type of measurement which may be partially overcome by including 'known standards'. This may be difficult in practice, but less so if the assessment is made from photographs which can be sorted prior to quantification.

Mechanical methods

A more objective approach can be made using mechanical methods. The most commonly used of these is replica profilometry (or surfometry). This can be done as a one-step or two-step procedure giving a negative and positive replica respectively (Figure 3.1).

REPLICA METHOD & DISADVANTAGES

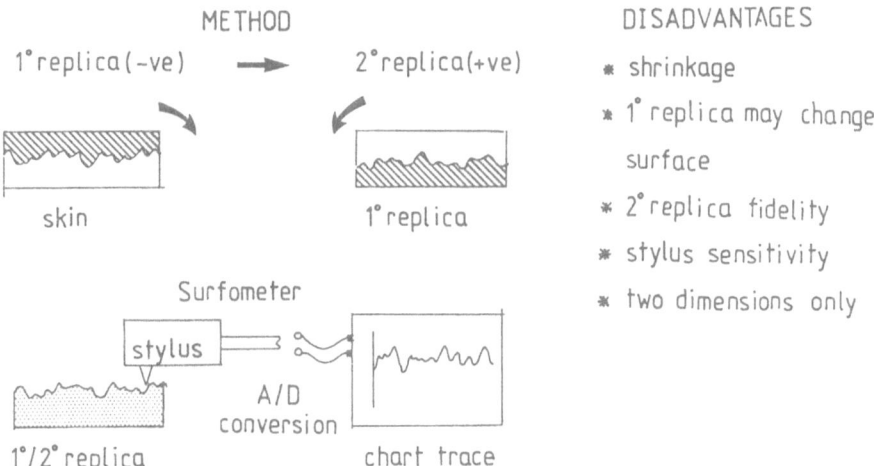

Figure 3.1 Diagrammatic representation of the replica method together with some disadvantages (see text for description)

The first stage is to apply a monomer and catalyst mixture to the skin surface and allow this to polymerize. The mixture used in our unit in Cardiff is silicone-rubber based, marketed as a dental impression material, Silflo (Flexico Developments Ltd., England). The impression of the skin surface can then be converted into a positive image by overlaying it with a styrene-polymer or epoxy resin that will faithfully replicate the original negative image. Alternatively, hydraulic cement has been used in a one-step procedure with the advantage that artefacts are limited to this single process[2]. The hardened final replica, whether positive or negative, can be measured by a profilometer. The principle of this is that the stylus is drawn across the replica and converts vertical displacement into a signal which can be output to a chart recorder or computer. The trace which is produced can be interpreted in various ways. The resolution is determined by the stylus tip diameter irrespective of the quality of the replica.

Figure 3.2 shows the profile of the skin before and after occlusive treatment with white soft paraffin for 30 minutes. Hydration produces swelling of the stratum corneum ironing out the small wrinkles and flattening the profile. The replica can also be observed by scanning electron microscopy and the small marks made by the profilometer stylus can sometimes be seen. In order to assess the profile, roughness parameters borrowed from the metallurgical industry have been adopted and applied to the trace generated from the replica. Table 3.1 summarizes these and their meaning.

SURFACE PROFILE CHANGES WITH WHITE SOFT PARAFFIN (W.S.P.) OCCLUSION. (Forearm site)

(a) Before

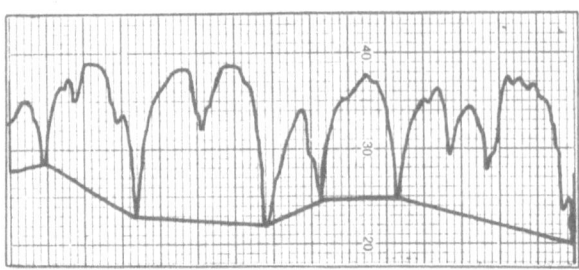

(b) After 1/2 h

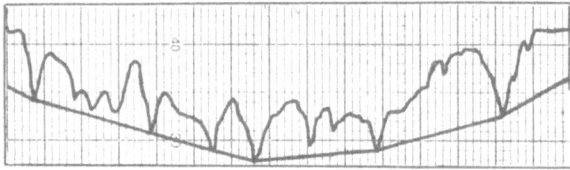

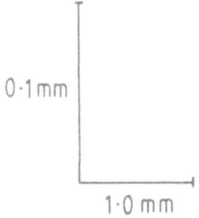

0·1mm

1·0 mm

Figure 3.2 The effect of application of white soft paraffin on skin surface profile

Table 3.1 Some roughness parameters used in assessing the skin surface after profilometry

R_a	Average roughness	Area under the trace per unit length
R_s	Profile length	Total profile length, per unit length
R_z	Mean peak height	Average of maximum peak height in defined sections of trace
R_t	Maximum peak height	Within a specified trace length
R_n	Number of peaks	Per unit length

The manner in which these values are calculated may vary from one establishment to another. One of the difficulties with this method is that the baseline is unknown, it being impossible to 'draw in' the base of the stratum corneum. Our own method of overcoming this is to join the major troughs and thus estimate the area under the curve R_a from this (see Figure 3.2). The resulting value can then be thought of as a measure of the volume of stratum corneum above the major troughs. Other methods calculate a mean profile height (mean voltage response from the profilometer) and R_a is then derived from the absolute area subtended either side of this mean value.

The trace produced by a profilometer is two dimensional. In our work we calculate mean values from multiple traces in the same direction. This produces an assessment of the roughness in one orientation. On some occasions it is necessary to assess roughness in the other, orthogonal direction. As an attempt to consider the whole three-dimensional surface of the skin, this has recently been superceded by making traces at steps across the replica automatically and storing the information[3]. This technique has produced a three-dimensional reconstruction of the surface and parameters which may be of use in comparing surface contour irrespective of the anisotropy that exists. These parameters are somewhat complex and cannot therefore be expounded here. However the 'real surface' - the ratio between the undulating surface and its two-dimensional projection - represents an easily understood measure of skin surface contour.

Optical methods

If mechanical methods represent an objective substitute for the human tactile assessment, the optical methods are attempts to make the surface appearance quantitative. In fact, there are two distinct approaches. One uses the replication techniques to provide the source of information, the other, photographic recording. Whilst the replication procedure mentioned above is used, it must be compared to a method which analyses scaliness at a finer level. Microscope slides, coated with adhesive, have been used to remove a sample of corneocytes from the surface of the skin, which are then submitted to image analysis to quantify the pattern and degree of corneocyte scaling[4,5]. These methods are based on the assumption that the pattern and distribution of corneocytes at the surface are dictated not only by corneocyte scaling, but also, if the initial sample is obtained with minimal pressure, by the distribution of the major features of the skin surface. In this respect the methods may represent an advance in being able to quantify the long and medium wavelength changes.

Quantification of the major skin patterns can also be obtained from silicone rubber or silastic replicas using optical methods. The first approach involves the use of an automatic focusing microscope which converts the change in focus to change in depth[6]. Sampling is carried out across the whole field of the replica and a three-dimensional image of the surface can be built up by automatic data acquisition. The method can detect gross changes in surface topography such as atrophy but the roughness parameter used may be insensitive to subtler alterations in contour. This is because the parameter, standard error of the plot of change in depth (focus) upon length of trace, is highly influenced by major skin features.

Corcuff et al.[7] have used the replica as a skin analogue and highlighted the relief with illumination from a shallow angle. Their image analysis system then quantifies the shadow, producing a measure of depth for the major skin features. However, the anisotropy is also accounted for by measuring the properties at several angles. In this way they have found the major and minor preferred axes of orientation of the surface features. In fact, by using the image analysis computer to the full they are able to search for these axes and record measurements solely from these aspects (Figure 3.3).

One of the problems associated with skin surface replicas is that they may influence the very physical properties that one is attempting to measure. Corneocytes - clumped or individual - may adhere to the replicating material. Uneven shrinkage of the replicating material or the secondary positive may also occur. It is for this reason that a completely non-invasive method has been developed, thus avoiding the flattening effect of the replicating material.

Photographic methods

Standardized macrophotographs have been used as a permanent source of skin image in Cardiff for some time[8]. Just as Corcuff et al. highlight the major skin features of replicas with shallow illumination, so in this method a photograph is taken from a standardized distance using a macro-lens. The flashgun is positioned 50 cm from the site at an angle of 25° to the horizontal. In this case all photographs are taken along the axis of the body site chosen. The photograph includes internal standards of reflectance and length which ensure the reproducibility of the process. The method assumes that the density of the silver grains is proportional to the reflectance of the surface, and that the latter is related in some way to skin surface contour.

The negative is scanned several times by a densitometer and assessed using the same roughness parameters used for replicas. Again there is no baseline and a moving average is calculated to serve as the point of reference to derive R_a, R_s, etc. (see Table 3.1). Results have been compared with those generated by replica profilometry and are in general agreement. However, the analysis of several lines across the profile ignores the three-dimensional anisotropy.

In an attempt to overcome this shortcoming and to use all the information available from the macrophotograph, we assessed the

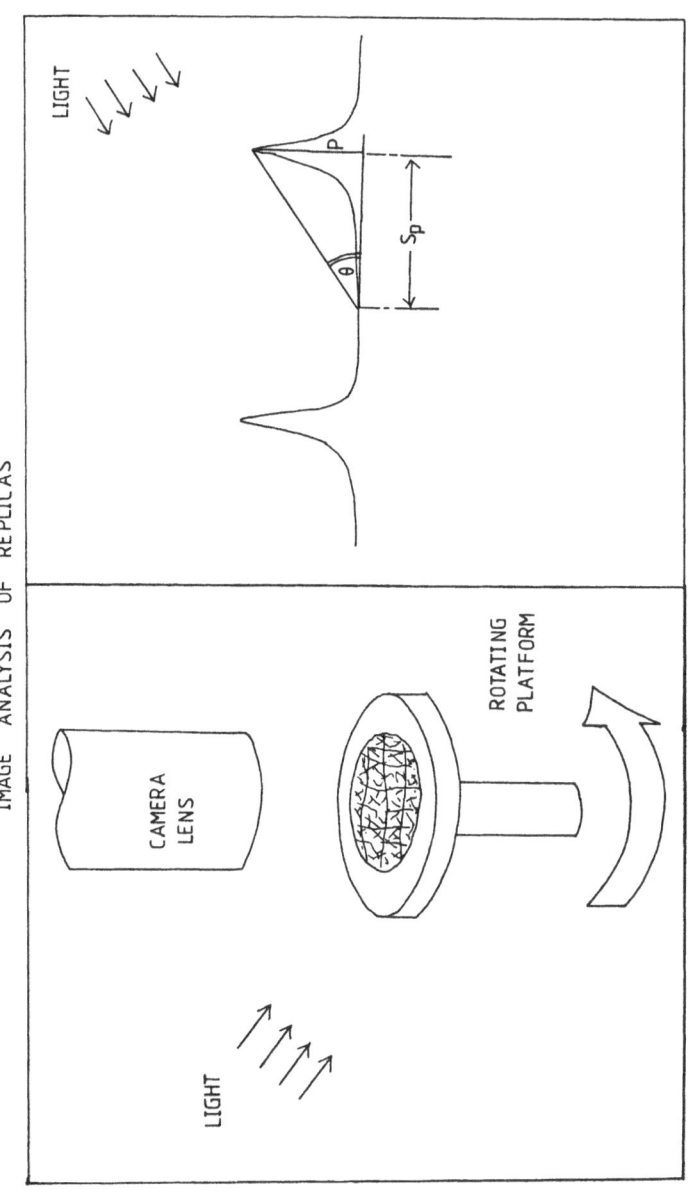

Figure 3.3 Image analysis of replicas. A light source applied at a given angle (θ) produces a shadow profile (S_p) which can be detected by the camera and interpreted by the image analyser. Profile height (P) can be derived trigonometrically

negatives by image analysis[9]. Again the negative was assessed densitometrically but this time the image analyser was programmed to step through the range of density intervals which, by calibration from the reflectance standards, were equivalent to steps of reflectance. At each step of reflectance, the area and intercept of those parts of greater reflectance than the present value could be derived. From this information, assuming that the greatest intercept value represents the maximum information, the mean width of the major features could be calculated and this converted to a value for mean height. Thus all the information was used from the whole area, but a three-dimensional value had not been derived.

This was achieved by summing all the perimeter measurements from each reflectance step and multiplying by the reflectance increment. This estimate - Reflective Surface Area - proved to be a less robust parameter, partly as a result of the reflectance increment, which varied between negatives. It was also a function of the image analyser resolution - 63 density steps - and may be improved upon with more sophisticated image processing prior to density measurement.

CONCLUSIONS

In summary, skin surface contour is a function of several aspects of stratum corneum and skin physical properties. Its contour also varies from site to site and as a function of age and sex. It also exhibits marked anisotropy. Measurement of skin contour allows assessment of many stratum corneum phenomena, from scaling to the emollient effects of applied materials. Objective methods of assessment allow several of the 'wavelength' components to be estimated with respect to their overall importance in the physical properties of the skin surface. In general, methods vary and should be chosen by consideration of time and cost-effectiveness together with invasiveness.

REFERENCES

1. Siegel, S. (1956). Non-Parametric Statistics for the Behavioural Sciences. (New York: McGraw Hill)
2. Gartstein, V. and Elsnau, W.H. (1985). Skin replicas using cement materials. Bioengineering and the Skin, 1(3), 287 (abstract)
3. Mignot, J., Chuard, M., Zahouani, H., Makki, S. and Agache, P. (1985). Microtopographical analysis of human skin surface. Bioengineering and the Skin, 1(2), 101
4. Spencer, T.S. and Seitz, J.C. (1985). Evaluation of corneocyte scaling with three different methods. Bioengineering and the Skin, 1(3), 253 (abstract)
5. Grove, G. and Grove, M. (1985). Objective assessment of skin surface scaliness through digital image processing of sticky slides. Bioengineering and the Skin, 1(3), 253 (abstract)
6. Gormley, D.E. (1985). Three dimensional optical micrometric analysis of casts of cutaneous surfaces. Bioengineering and the Skin, 1(2), 81
7. Corcuff, P., Chatenay, F. and Leveque, J-L. (1984). A fully automated system to study skin surface patterns. Int. J. Cosmetic Sci., 6, 167
8. Marshall, R.J. and Marks, R. (1983). Assessment of the skin surface by scanning densitometry of macrophotographs. Clin. Exp. Dermatol., 8, 121
9. Barton, S.P., Marshall, R.J. and Marks, R. (1987). A novel method for assessing skin surface topography. Bioengineering and the Skin, 3, 93

Chapter 4

Skin imaging: a comparison of available techniques

P A Payne

INTRODUCTION

In addressing the subject of skin imaging in this chapter, imaging will be regarded as a technique for obtaining structural data in a cross-sectional sense, in other words, a measurement technique that will also provide the user with a pictorial representation of the skin, similar to that obtained by excision of a small piece of skin and the study of this skin section under a low power microscope. Using this interpretation of the word 'imaging' it will be seen that there is a close link between the measurement technique for skin thickness and the more elaborate method of using such a technique for imaging. This relationship is dealt with in some detail later.

A further reason for developing methods of skin thickness measurement and skin imaging based on the use of probing energies such as ultrasound or electromagnetic waves is that in a comparative sense, these are non-invasive techniques. In the sense that any measurement must disturb the measurand to some extent, then there is no non-invasive method. However, if one compares the degree of damage done to the tissue under investigation using ultrasound, then this is of a far smaller degree than the damage induced by the use of skin biopsy in order to accomplish the same end. In fact, ultrasound has so far been found to produce no detectable biological changes in the biological tissue under investigation when the power levels are kept to recommended maxima. In contrast, X-ray energy is known to be a potential cause of neoplastic change and may be described as somewhat more invasive than ultrasound.

SKIN THICKNESS MEASUREMENTS

We can separate skin thickness measurement techniques into two major types, the first based on the removal of a sample of skin and its subsequent examination using the light microscope following a variety of staining techniques[1]. The second area relates to in vivo measurements in which the skin thickness data are obtained without incurring damage to the integrity of the skin.

A further division in the case of the in vivo techniques is between those using electromagnetic energy, such as X-rays[2] or radio waves (the basis of magnetic resonance imaging, for example) and those using mechanical energy, such as ultrasound[3]. The skin 'pinch' or skin fold approach[4] to in vivo measurement must be seen as a separate category in terms of these divisions.

METHODS

In vitro

The use of a conventional light microscope with low magnification (up to 100 times) is a relatively simple technique based on the use of a variety of organic dyes to provide the necessary contrast between various parts of the skin and the subcutaneous fat[5].

The use of different forms of energy, e.g. electromagnetic waves or ultrasound suggests that we should consider whether data obtained using these different forms of energy will give rise to measurements that can be directly compared. In obtaining measurements on whole skin thickness we rely on detecting an interface between the base of the dermis and the subcutaneous fat. This junction is easy to find using the light microscope and it is likely that the same interface is distinguished by ultrasound as well (see later). However, when we wish to look at more subtle interfaces, such as that between the papillary dermis and the reticular dermis, we cannot guarantee that light microscopy will give exactly the same interface position data as that obtained using reflections of ultrasound energy generated by very small changes in acoustic properties. When we compare the ultrasound and X-ray methods, similar arguments apply and these comparisons are probably even more suspect. Added complications arise due to small changes in propagation velocity using ultrasound which must be properly accounted for if measurements on the various layers of skin are to be reliably determined. Further discussion of these comparisons will be provided later.

It is, of course, possible to employ xeroradiography and ultrasound to determine the thickness of skin tissue obtained at biopsy and, provided sufficient attention is paid to the effects of temperature, humidity and resting tension, the in vitro approach can be used effectively to build up the large body of data required to establish normal variation between subjects and between body sites.

Radiological techniques

Techniques of skin thickness measurement based on X-rays have been employed for some time[6] and modified more recently[7] and applied to studies of dermal atrophy[8]. The method as described by Marks et al.[8] employs tangential X-rays at 120 kV which are directed at the flexor aspect of the forearm. It is also necessary to flatten the region of skin to be examined. Xerox paper is employed rather than X-ray film giving a better, more easily examined image. A permanent positive image is produced from which thickness measurements, using optical methods, can be obtained.

Disadvantages of the xeroradiographic method[7,9] are that it can only be employed on the forearm and also requires large areas of skin. Further, the ionizing form of radiation employed must raise doubts about its prolonged use for serial studies. It does, however, compare favourably with other methods in terms of accuracy and resolution[9].

Ultrasound

At an International Symposium on Recent Advances in Ultrasound Diagnosis held in Dubrovnik in October 1977, Rukavina and Mohar presented some work on ultrasonic diagnosis of skin and subcutaneous tissue. This was subsequently published in 1979[10]. Although they were mostly concerned with diagnosis of subcutaneous lesions, their work probably represents the first report on the use of ultrasound in dermatology. The work was based on the use of a B-scan technique which provides a cross-sectional image and which is dealt with later in this chapter.

The first report on the use of A-scan techniques, designed to produce simple thickness measurements, is contained in the paper by Alexander and Miller[11]. Since this paper was published in 1979, there has been a steady growth in the amount of interest shown in the use of ultrasound for dermatology and in a few centres the technique has become a routine clinical measurement.

The physical basis for medical ultrasound

Ultrasound has been recognized for more than 100 years, but it was confined to research laboratories for most of this period because of the difficulties associated with generating and receiving ultrasonic signals. These difficulties were largely overcome with the advent of suitable transducer materials based on a range of ceramic composites and it is these materials that are the foundation for almost all current medical ultrasound[3].

Skin thickness measurements are simply obtained using the ultrasound pulse echo method. This is shown diagrammatically in Figures 4.1 and 4.2. Figure 4.1 shows the manner in which the signals are conveyed to and from the skin and Figure 4.2 illustrates very simply the layout of a pulse echo A-scan instrument.

It is tempting to believe that existing ultrasonic scanners can be applied to dermatological problems. This, however, turns out not to be the most effective route. Skin has structural differences compared with most other tissue successfully studied using ultrasound which makes it necessary to design a 'skin thickness meter' to specifically satisfy these requirements. The ultrasonic frequency at which such a meter must work is, of necessity, relatively high compared with most other medical applications. This is because the wavelength (the reciprocal of frequency) is the major determinant of resolution in skin thickness measurement. The skin is approximately 1-4.5 mm thick and if we are to resolve small changes in skin thickness (less than 0.1 mm) then we require a wavelength of about this order. The relationship between wavelength and

33

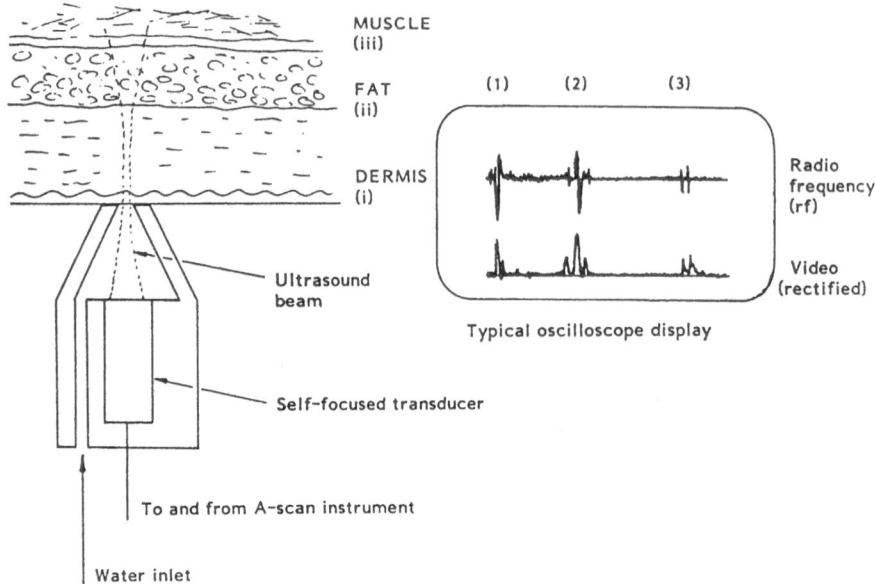

Figure 4.1   Pulse echo, A-scan arrangement showing transducer, stand-off and oscilloscope display. Echo (1) corresponds to region (i), i.e. stratum corneum/water interface. Echo (2) corresponds to region (ii), i.e. dermis/fat interface. Echo (3) corresponds to region (iii), i.e. fat/muscle fascia interface

frequency is given by the expression $c = f\lambda$, where c is the characteristic ultrasonic velocity (ms^{-1}) in the tissue under consideration, f the ultrasonic frequency (Hz) and λ the wavelength (m). From this we can see that for a wavelength of 0.1 mm and assuming a tissue velocity of 1500 m/s for convenience, we obtain an ultrasonic frequency of 15 MHz. It is no coincidence, therefore, that the transducer employed for the work of Alexander and Miller[11] was designed to operate at 15 MHz. All this is based on two major assumptions:

1.   The ultrasonic velocity quoted above applies to skin. This is a figure derived from work reported by Daly and Wheeler[12] and was performed on oral soft tissue. The exact figure that they published was 1518 m/s. This has been subsequently misquoted in various later papers and one can often find the figure of 1580 m/s employed for the velocity in skin, but using the Daly and Wheeler paper as the justification for this. The first thing to note is that the work of Daly and Wheeler was based on oral soft tissue, which is not necessarily the same as skin ultrasonically. It was also performed on samples of tissue that had been removed at postmortem and fixed, which might change the velocity figure quite substantially. There has been much further work to determine the velocity of ultrasound in skin and it appears that an average figure through the epidermis and

34

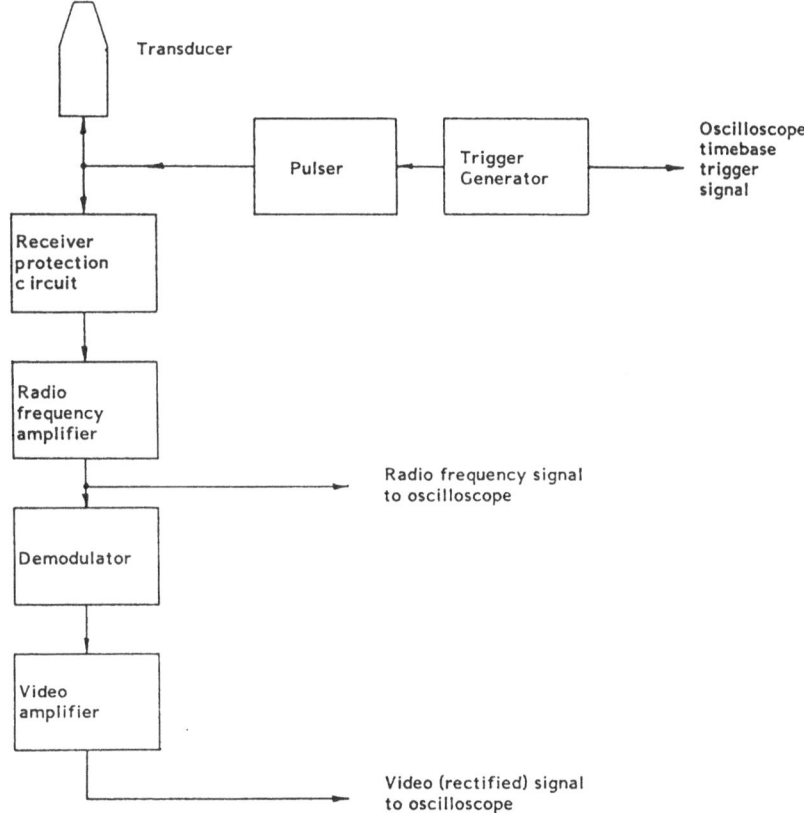

Figure 4.2 Simplified block diagram of A-scan pulse echo instrumentation

dermis of around 1600 m/s may well be the best compromise[13]. No doubt there are many other factors that can change the velocity of ultrasound in skin, including pathological states and perhaps regional variation around the body. These measurements have yet to be made, but the figure quoted (1600 m/s) would appear to be a very satisfactory compromise.

2. The second assumption is that if we discuss ultrasound frequencies (in this case 15 MHz) then we can indeed associate the corresponding wavelength (0.1 mm) with the attainable resolution. This is only true if the frequency quoted is the centre frequency of a wide band transducer. The concept that we are dealing with is illustrated in Figure 4.3. In Figure 4.3(a) a narrow band transducer characteristic is shown by means of a graph of its output against frequency. The corresponding shape of the signal that would be obtained from such a transducer as an acoustic waveform, that is a graph of output against time and which is the signal actually dealt with in ultrasonic measurements

35

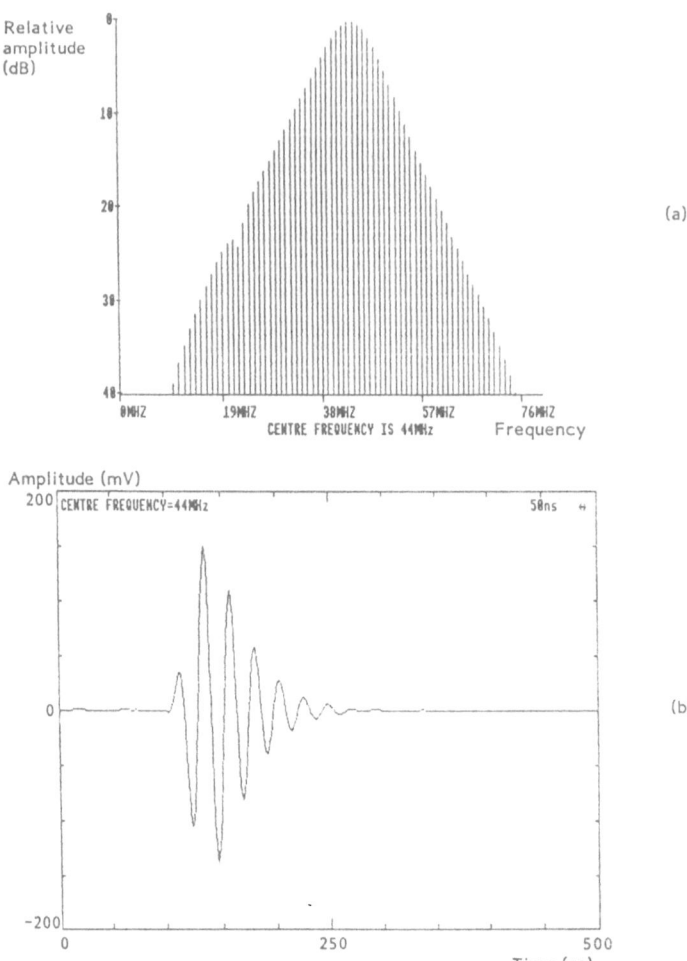

Figure 4.3 Characteristic frequency and time domain performance for a narrow band transducer operating in the pulse echo mode. (a) Typical narrow band transducer frequency spectrum having a 44 MHz centre frequency and 45% bandwidth (at -10 dB points); (b) echo pulse (obtained from a plane target) from which spectral data given in (a) above was obtained; (c) typical wide band transducer frequency spectrum having a 38 MHz centre frequency and 147% bandwidth (at -10 dB points); (d) echo pulse (obtained from a plane target) from which spectral data given in (a) above was obtained

systems, is shown in Figure 4.3(b). Contrast this with a wide band transducer, having the same centre frequency, the response for which is shown in Figure 4.3(c) and the time waveform is Figure 4.3(d). As can be seen in comparing Figure 4.3(b) with (d), the wide band transducer produces a time response, the duration of which is very much shorter. Now, since time and distance in making thickness measurements within the skin are interchangeable, it is clear that the shorter the

36

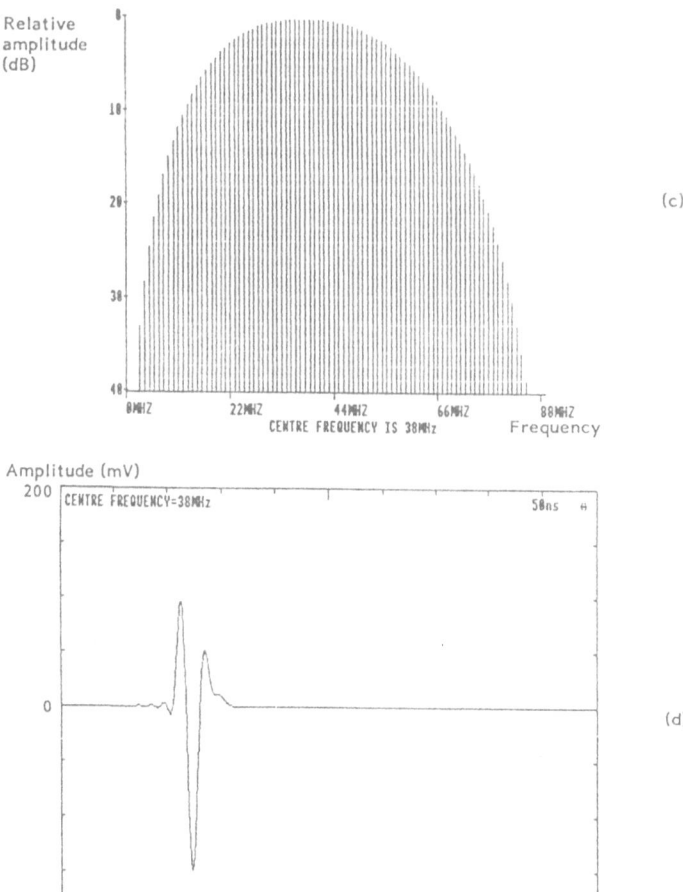

Figure 4.3 (continued)

duration of the time waveform for a given transducer, the better it will be in terms of resolution. It is for this reason that considerable effort has been put into the design and construction of wide band high frequency transducers for use in dermatological ultrasound.

The discussion so far concerning resolution has concentrated on the axial resolution, that is, the depth or thickness resolution obtained during measurement. We must also concern ourselves with the lateral resolution obtained and this is primarily defined by the characteristic shape of the ultrasound beam projected from the transducer. A transducer can be constructed with either focused or non-focused characteristics. The non-focused, flat transducer will have a beam profile in the useful region approximately equal to the cross-section of the transducer element. Typically, small transducers used in dermatology will be of the order of 1 cm in diameter and, therefore, the signals obtained will represent an average thickness reading over such a cross-sectional area. If, however, a focused transducer is employed, we can obtain a focal region of less than 1 mm in diameter, if necessary, and those devices will give rise to 'spot' measurements of skin thickness. Both approaches have advantages and disadvantages depending on the particular investigations.

Typical A-scan data

Figure 4.4 shows an A-scan echo pattern received from normal inner forearm skin, and as can be seen, the first major echo is as a result of the coupling medium/epidermis junction, the second major echo results from the dermis/subcutaneous junction and the third major echo, usually present, results from the interface between the subcutaneous fat and muscle fascia. Within the region enclosed by the first and second major echoes are smaller echoes which arise from the structure within the epidermis and dermis. A characteristic relatively echo-free region is seen from the subcutaneous fat region which is often useful to aid in the interpretation of such an image. The data shown in Figure 4.4 were obtained using a transducer based on polymer materials[14] and broad bandwidth transducers of this type appear to be a very useful development.

Applications

Dermal atrophy is a well known side-effect occurring during treatment by corticosteroids and it is important to monitor their skin thinning effects. Previous studies have compared xeroradiographic and ultrasonic methods for measuring the thinning activity and have shown extremely good correlation between the two groups of data. A reduction in the dermal thickness of the order of 4-5% is detectable as early as 2 days after treatment with very potent corticosteroids. Following a 7 week treatment regime, the dermal thickness was found to have returned to within 91-96% of the pretreatment values after a further 4 weeks[9].

Dermal atrophy can also occur due to radiation therapy and the xeroradiographic or ultrasound technique may be used to monitor and chart the progress of such atrophy. Much work on this effect has been performed by Hamlet et al.[15] and in this they have also used ultrasound for skin thickness measurements.

Another area in which skin thickness measurements are of importance is that of burn damaged skin. Skin affected by burns can develop thick scar tissue and a variety of treatment techniques are employed to reduce such scar tissue. Pressure garments appear

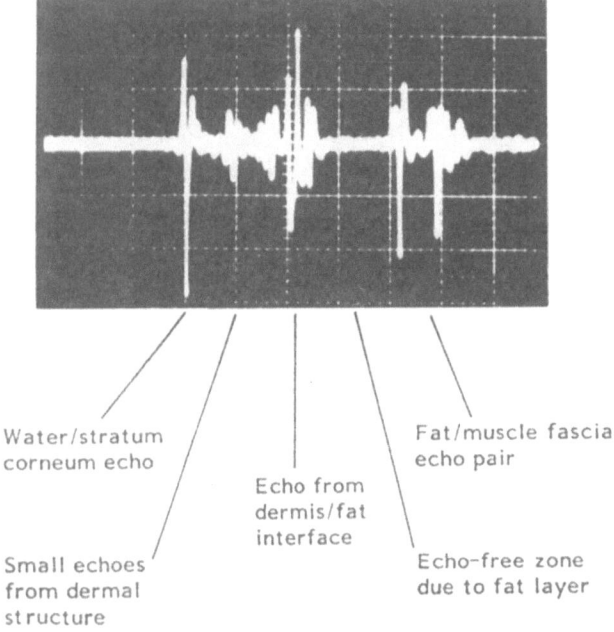

Water/stratum
corneum echo

Echo from
dermis/fat
interface

Fat/muscle fascia
echo pair

Small echoes
from dermal
structure

Echo-free zone
due to fat layer

Scales: Vertical   100 mV per division
         Horizontal 500 ns per division

Figure 4.4 Ultrasound A-scan pattern from normal human skin (inner forearm)

to be of use in reducing scar tissue formation and the ultrasound skin thickness technique has been found to give an indication of the efficacy of pressure garment treatment[16]. There are difficulties in that scar can produce echoes which are difficult to interpret and very thick tissue can totally absorb the ultrasound energy preventing detection of echos from the bottom of the scar tissue. These problems, however, can be overcome by appropriate choice of equipment. A similar measurement made using the xeroradiographic technique would require high X-ray energies and this and the many successive measurements would tend to rule out this approach.

In a series of papers[17-19] Serup has investigated the use of ultrasound thickness measurements to evaluate a variety of conditions affecting the thickness of skin. He uses a 15 MHz transducer which is fitted with a gelatin stand-off which is more convenient than the water stand-off often employed by others. Results of his work in investigating the effect of various concentrations of histamine applied as a skin prick test are given[18]. He uses a system which displays the ultrasonic echo as a unipolar signal. This is achieved by rectifying the radiofrequency signal and some workers have claimed that these data are easier to interpret.

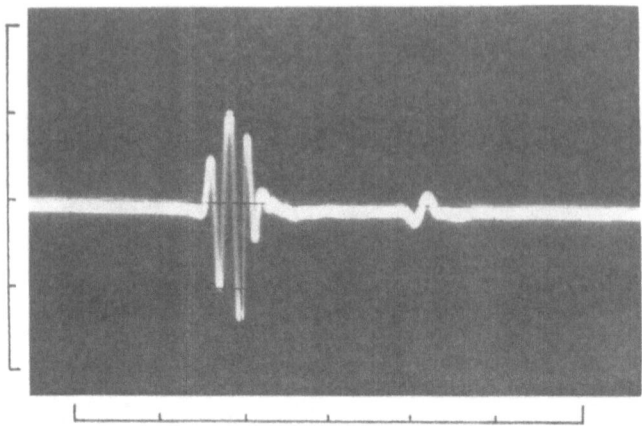

Scales: Vertical   0.5 V per division
       Horizontal 0.2 µs per division

Figure 4.5 Ultrasound A-scan of human thumbnail (from Finlay et al.[20])

Certainly they are far less complex than the radiofrequency signals.
His results from measurements in psoriasis and morphoea tend to
confirm the ability of the ultrasound A-scan method to provide
useful indications of the change in thickness due to various
pathological conditions.

Recently interest has arisen in the use of the ultrasonic A-scan
method to measure thickness changes in human nail. A study of
normal human finger nails has been undertaken by Finlay et al.[20]
and in Figure 4.5 a typical result from a normal human thumb nail
is shown. This was obtained at a distal position on the thumb nail
using a 20 MHz ultrasound A-scan system. Finlay and his colleagues
have obtained preliminary data for normal nail thickness and have
compared the ultrasonic data with figures obtained from a
micrometer. These comparisons indicate that the ultrasonic technique
is highly reliable and can be used to assess objectively the effects
of disease, topical applications and systemic drugs such as
retinoids. They have pointed out that, although nail thickness can
be measured at the free edge of the nail, there is variability across
the nail plate and that such distal thickness measurements may take
many months to reflect changes due to proximal nail growth
variations which are themselves caused by disease, etc.

Ultrasound B-scanning of skin

The physical principles upon which the B-scan is based are identical to those already described in the section on ultrasound A-scanning above. The difference is in the method in which the data are collected and displayed.

Two major divisions exist generally in this type of work. The first is based on the mechanical scanning of a single element transducer and the second on the use of some form of transducer array in which the movement of the ultrasonic beam is achieved electronically. Due to the resolution requirements imposed by the skin, the second alternative, that of ultrasonic array scanning, is not acceptable. This is because the resolution requirements dictate corresponding requirements for array geometry and electronic systems that are technologically not feasible at present. However, if the clinical requirements associated with B-scanning are somewhat relaxed and the structures under investigation are of larger dimension than those associated with normal skin, such as in the case of benign or malignant tumours just under the skin, then available transducer array technology may be applicable[10].

Most of the published B-scan data have been obtained using single element transducers in conjunction with mechanical scanning and Figure 4.6 shows the manner in which such images are obtained.

The earliest work on ultrasound and skin was performed with a standard medical B-scanner[10]. However, the first high resolution skin images of a cross-sectional nature were obtained by Payne et al. in 1981[21]. A result typical of those obtainable in this fashion is given in Figure 4.6(b). More recently, attention has been given to the deficiencies of this simple approach, the major limitation of which is imposed by the low bandwidth of the storage oscilloscopes employed (perhaps only some 10 MHz). This is to be contrasted with the bandwidth of good plastic film transducers, typically some 20-25 MHz. The loss of overall measurement bandwidth substantially reduces the image quality possible. A method for retaining full measurement bandwidth is available by adopting an approach based on capturing the echo data in a digital fashion followed by storage, manipulation and eventual display of the stored data. In this way, bandwidth is traded for processing time and the image is no longer produced in real time. The potential for very high resolution B-scans is available from this approach.

Magnetic resonance imaging (MRI) of skin

The use of nuclear magnetic resonance (NMR) as an imaging technique is a recent innovation which has aroused considerable interest since, unlike X-ray methods, the NMR approach provides excellent details of soft tissue structure. In addition, the method is thought to be less invasive or hazardous than X-ray methods, although long-term effects are as yet uncertain.

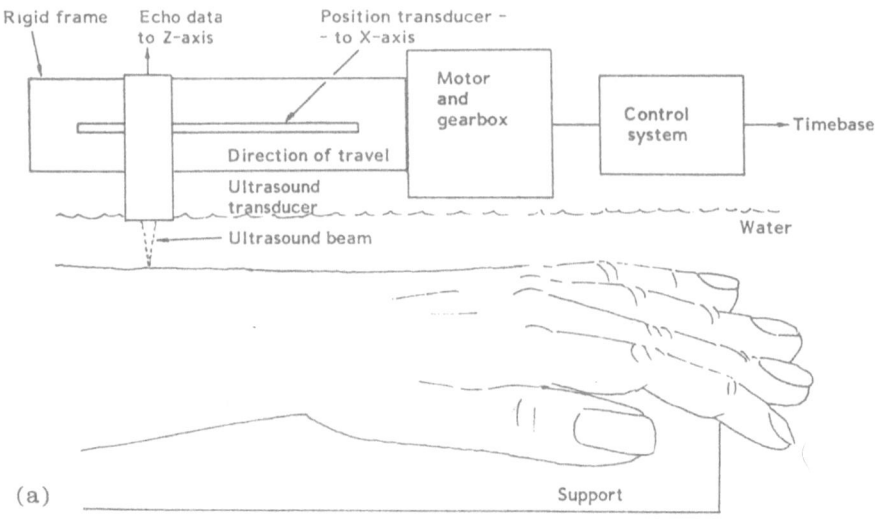

(a)

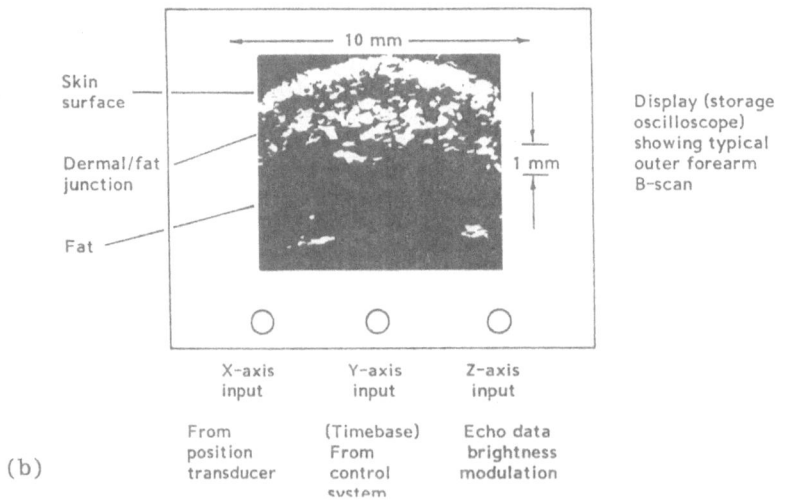

(b)

Figure 4.6 Mechanical B-scan ultrasound system. (a) B-scan ultrasound system; (b) typical results from normal outer forearm skin

Magnetic resonance imaging has developed recently from the well established use of NMR as an analytical spectroscopic technique. NMR is dependent on the nuclear spin which generates a magnetic movement and those nuclei having a zero spin are not amenable to this measurement method. The effects are induced by placing a sample in a magnetic field which is then disturbed by a second oscillating field. The signal detected is due to the effects of the disturbances in the nuclei which can be arranged to generate voltages in a receiver coil.

Methods for converting this measurement into an imaging technique have been developed. The extension of this method to imaging of skin has been under consideration for some time.

Applications of cross-sectional imaging

The major reason for turning to the more complex mode of B-scanning for employing ultrasound on the skin is that the cross-sectional image so obtained is far easier to understand than A-scan data in the presence of disease. Examples of this include malignant tumours such as melanoma, squamous cell carcinoma and basal cell carcinoma. In each case the change in the pattern of A-scan echoes is often so complex that measurements of dimensions are difficult. However, if a B-scan is undertaken in such conditions, the appearance of the tumour is very clearly indicated and a subsequent A-scan measurement can then be undertaken to obtain, for example, the depth of the tumour and possibly even some information concerning its classification. The B-scan can also indicate the extent in area of the tumour under the skin. For some while now a group led by Dr E W Breitbart of the Skin Department at the University of Hamburg, West Germany, has been employing these techniques[22-24].

This same group has, in addition, combined the B-scanning technique with a method for examining the elastic characteristics of skin (the so-called M-mode) and this provides them with a simple in vivo determination of the changes in dimension of the skin under mechanical deformation[23].

Further work employing B-scan ultrasound has been undertaken by a group in the Department of Dermatology at the University of Ehime School of Medicine in Japan. They have investigated benign and malignant lesions in lymph nodes and have looked at the possibility of using ultrasound attenuation methods to obtain diagnosis[25,26].

CONCLUSIONS

Measurement of skin thickness plays an important role in a number of clinical and research activities within dermatology and techniques based on simple A-scan ultrasound have been found to be concise and accurate. One major advantage of the ultrasound A-scan method is that it can be used successively on a particular area of skin in order to track changes due to a disease process or due to treatment.

A difficulty associated with the A-scan technique is that the data can become confusing and the B-scan method has been adopted to cope with this. Ultrasound B-scans of a high resolution nature sufficient to give good measurements of the various layers of the skin are a relatively recent innovation and not a great deal of clinical experience has yet been gained. As this experience is built up it is expected that the B-scan method will become increasingly important.

The B-scan technique, as conventionally applied with a storage oscilloscope, does have severe limitations in terms of the potential resolution obtainable and the solution to this has been to turn to B-scans with a digital image capability. This improves the resolution considerably, but the technique is more expensive and slower.

Even more recent is the advent of magnetic resonance imaging of skin. This provides an interesting comparison with ultrasound B-scans and the combined application of these two imaging techniques may well be the ultimate answer to the diagnosis of small lesions within the skin. It would, however, be a somewhat expensive solution.

REFERENCES

1. Shuster, S., Black, M.M. and McVitie, E. (1975). The influence of age and sex on skin thickness, skin collagen and density. Br. J. Dermatol., **93**, 639
2. Tan, C.Y., Marks, R., Roberts, E. and Guibarra, E. (1981). Xeroradiographic and ultrasound techniques in the assessment of skin disorder. In Marks, R. and Payne, P.A. (eds.) Bioengineering and the Skin. p. 215. (Lancaster: MTP Press)
3. Payne, P.A. (1985). Medical and industrial applications of high resolution ultrasound. J. Phys. E. Sci. Instrum., **16**, 465
4. Tanner, J.M. and Whitehouse, R.H. (1955). The Harpenden skinfold caliper. Am. J. Physical Anthropology, **13**, 743
5. Lapiere, Ch.M. (1979). Techniques for investigating collagen in pathology. In Marks, R. (ed.) Investigative Techniques in Dermatology. p. 191. (Oxford: Blackwell Scientific Publications)
6. Shephard, R.H. and Meema, H.E. (1967). Skin thickness in endocrine disease. Ann. Intern. Med., **66**, 531
7. Black, M.M. (1969). A modified radiographic method for measuring skin thickness. Br. J. Dermatol., **81**, 661
8. Marks, R., Dykes, P.J. and Roberts, E. (1975). The measurement of corticosteroid induced dermal atrophy by a radiological method. Arch. Dermatol. Res., **253**, 93
9. Tan, C.Y., Marks, R. and Payne, P.A. (1981). Comparison of xeroradiographic and ultrasound detection of corticosteroid induced dermal thinning. J. Invest. Dermatol., **76**, 126
10. Rukavina, B. and Mohar, N. (1979). An approach of ultrasound diagnostic techniques in the skin and subcutaneous tissue. Dermatologica, **158**, 81
11. Alexander, H. and Miller, D.L. (1979). Determining skin thickness with pulsed ultrasound. J. Invest. Dermatol., **72**, 17
12. Daly, C.H. and Wheeler, J.B. (1971). The use of ultrasonic thickness measurements in the clinical evaluation of soft tissue. Int. Dental. J., **21**, 418
13. Escoffier, C., Querleux, B., Rigal, J. de and Leveque, J.L. (1986). In vitro study of the velocity of ultrasound in the skin. Bioeng. Skin, **1**, 87
14. Edwards, C. (1984). The use of high frequency ultrasound to study dimensions and properties of skin. PhD Thesis. University of Manchester Faculty of Technology
15. Hamlet, R., Rezvani, M. and Hopewell, J.W. (1986). Ultrasound measurement of atrophy in pig skin following X- or β-irradiation. Bioeng. Skin, **2**, 49
16. Clarke, J.A. (1985). Ultrasound thickness measurements of burn scar tissue. Bioeng. Skin, **1**, 71
17. Serup, J. (1984). Non-invasive quantification of psoriasis plaques - measurement of skin thickness with 15 MHz pulsed ultrasound. Clin. Exp. Dermatol., **9**, 502
18. Serup, J. (1984). Diameter, thickness, area and volume of skin-prick histamine weals. Allergy, **39**, 359
19. Serup, J. (1984). Localized scleroderma (morphoea): thickness of sclerotic plaques as measured by 15 MHz pulsed ultrasound. Acta Dermatol. Venereol., **64**, 214
20. Finlay, A.Y., Moseley, H. and Duggan, T.C. (1986). Nail thickness by ultrasound. Bioeng. Skin, **2**, 181
21. Payne, P.A., Grove, G.L., Alexander, H., Quilliam, R.M. and Miller, D.L. (1981). Cross-sectional ultrasonic scanning of the skin using plastic film transducers. Bioeng. Skin Newsletter, **3**, 214

22. Breitbart, E.W. and Rehpenning, W. (1985). Ultrasonic diagnosis of malignant tumours of the skin. Bioeng. Skin, 1, 76

23. Breitbart, E.W., Rehpenning, W., Hicks, R. and Dyson, E. (1985). In vivo investigations of the skin, its structure and elasticity with high frequency ultrasound. Bioeng. Skin, 1, 231

24. Breitbart, E.W., Rehpenning, W., Hicks, R. and Dyson, E. (1985). Ultrasound diagnosis of malignant tumours of the skin, especially malignant melanoma. Bioeng. Skin, 1, 284

25. Miyauchi, S., Murakami, S. and Miki, Y. (1985). Echographic studies on superficial lymphadenopathies. Bioeng. Skin, 1, 230

26. Murakami, S., Miyauchi, S. and Miki, Y. (1985). A new 20 MHz ultrasonic scanner for dermatological use. Bioeng. Skin, 1, 289

Chapter 5

Making sense of numbers from the skin

M F Corbett

INTRODUCTION

Before reporting the findings from a study, the data which have been so carefully collected must be summarized, and appropriate analyses made. A choice must be made from a considerable variety of methods of summarizing data. Ways of exploring and examining the data before choosing the summary and analysis are considered here.

DATA STRUCTURE

A well-chosen method of data summary is one which gives a representative central value and also indicates how widely dispersed the observations are. For example, if the maximum diameters of skin lesions, measured in millimetres (an interval scale of measurement), are symmetrically distributed with the bulk of observations clustered around the middle of the range and with maximum and minimum values approximately equal distances from the middle, a set of such observations could be summarized by calculating the mean value and the standard deviation of the values in the set. The mean and standard deviation, however, are not always the best choice for summarizing a particular set of observations; they are not always appropriate and they are easily disturbed by a few unusual observations in the set. The best choice of summary takes account of the scale of measurement used in making the observations and also of their distribution.

Interrelationships in a set of observations are shown by its data structure. Understanding the structure of the data includes deciding what constitutes the fundamental experimental unit, how these units are grouped, and precisely what are the variables, and how they are measured. An example of data structure is shown in Table 5.1. It shows surfometry measurements made from skin surface replicas obtained before and also after stretching forearm skin with an extensometer. The observations show the length of a traced line drawn by the surfometer as it follows the surface of the skin replica between two points a standard distance apart. From the table it is clear that six individuals were used for the measurements. A replica was made from the area before any extension of skin was done, followed by further replicas made after extensions of 5 and 10 mm. Surfometry tracings were made from each replica along lines both parallel to the direction of extension and perpendicular to this direction. The rows represent individuals, each one of whom had three skin replicas made from his forearm, while the columns show two different sets of observations, measured at right angles to each other. Thus the data structure shows both the nature and number of the measurements and the groupings and classification of the individuals on whom the measurements were made[1]. The grouping of individuals is specially important because grouping should be considered in the analysis, since many statistical procedures are sensitive to lack of independence. Thus the method of analysis of observations made within individuals (repeated measurements on one individual) must be one which does not assume that the observations are completely independent of each other.

Table 5.1 Line length from skin surface replica before and after extensometry (mm)

Extension (mm)	Parallel			Perpendicular		
	0	5	10	0	5	10
AB	581	369	317	554	608	779
CD	560	499	271	580	673	718
EF	536	369	370	666	771	604
GH	534	399	322	569	692	669
IJ	525	370	370	585	628	633
KL	719	538	292	496	651	880

QUALITY CHECKS

Having chosen the preferred method of summary, but before it is done, it is useful to check the quality of the data which have been collected. Simple quality checks include:

1. An inspection for values which are inconsistent or in conflict with prior information about the range of values likely to be observed. The maximum and mimimum values of each variable are useful because they may draw attention to one or more atypical values.

2. The frequency distribution of each main variable. This graphical technique may show one or more discrepant observations. It is also useful to determine whether the distribution appears to be symmetrical or skewed, because the method of summary may not be resistant to skewness of the observations - a problem which occurs quite often in practice. However, if it has to be performed by hand, constructing the plot can be laborious.

3. Outlying or discrepant observations clearly shown in a scatter plot of pairs of observations (if this is appropriate).

4. Consideration of the method of collection of the data is valuable as there may be indications of serious bias such as quantitative differences between the measurements made by different observers.

5. A common source of confusion in writing down observations is the lack of a clear distinction between a measurement value of zero and a zero put into the data to denote that an observation was not made. It is worthwhile to check the symbol used to identify a missing value. In good quality data it is essential that this distinction is unequivocal.

PRELIMINARY ANALYSIS

To avoid commonly made mistakes in the definitive analysis, this should be preceded by preliminary analysis, an exploratory examination of the data which can be combined with quality checking. Preliminary analysis is also an opportunity to review the data structure and to make sure that the structure will be correctly reflected in the methods employed for definitive analysis.

THE STEM-AND-LEAF DISPLAY

This simple graphical method of exploratory data analysis is a good beginning for preliminary analysis. It is easy to do by hand, but informative, and has also by now been incorporated in some of the commonly available statistical packages; for example, it is featured in both Minitab and SPSS[X]. The technique and the name, 'stem-and-leaf display', is due to J W Tukey[2]. Table 5.2 shows the area of experimental lesions measured from biopsies of treated skin in guinea pigs. The data are shown again in Figure 5.1 as a stem-and-leaf display. The first observation, 7.3, appears in the stem-and-leaf display as the second of two digits opposite the figure 7 in the upper part of the display. The display is constructed by choosing a suitable pair of digits in the data, in this example the ones digit and the tens digit. Each data value is then split between these digits to form a stem and a leaf:

observation	split	stem	and	leaf
7.3	7/3	7	and	3

In the simplest form of display, one line is allocated for each stem. The leaf, the next digit, of each value is written down on the line corresponding to its stem. Use only one digit for the leaf and truncate, rather than round off, observations - one of the virtues of the stem-and-leaf display is that it is relatively easy to identify each value after plotting. Thus, the place reached in plotting will not be lost after an interruption, and any mistake can easily be identified and put right.

49

Table 5.2 Area of inflammation (mm^2)

7.3	6.8	3.2	4.2	11.6	5.1	11.3	3.6
7.2	2.8	10.6	2.5	12.7	4.8	14.2	6.2
5.9	8.9	5.1	5.4	4.9	10.9	4.7	2.9

Area of inflammation (mm^2)
unit = 0.1 mm^2

```
 2 | 589
 3 | 26
 4 | 2789
 5 | 1149
 6 | 28
 7 | 23
 8 | 9
 9 |
10 | 69
11 | 36
12 | 7
13 |
14 | 2
```

n = 24

```
M 12.5 |        5.65
F  6.5 | 4.45           9.75
     1 | 2.5            14.2
```

Figure 5.1 Stem-and-leaf display and letter display data from Table 5.2

Once the observations have been set out in a stem-and-leaf display, they are almost sorted. As there are usually relatively few leaves on each stem it is a simple matter to rearrange them in order. At once the extreme values, here 2.5 and 14.2, can be identified. Each observation in the ordered array has a rank. The count up from the smallest value is its upward rank while the count downward from the largest value is its downward rank. The smaller of these two ranks is the 'depth' of the observation, for example, the most extreme values have a depth of 1.

It is easy to find the median in an ordered array of observations. The median of an odd number of observations is the middle number, but if n, the number of observations, is even, the median is the average of the two middle observations. When there are n observations, the median has depth (n+1)/2 - a whole number if n is odd, but not when n is even. To find the median it is only necessary to count in from either end of the array as far as indicated by the depth. Thus in Figure 5.1, n is 24 so the depth of the median is 12.5. Counting from either the smallest or the largest end, the median is the average of the 12th and the 13th observations, 5.65.

Below the stem-and-leaf display in Figure 5.1 is a 'letter-value' display showing some summarizing values. The letter 'M' stands for the median. Next to it is its depth, and in the box is the median itself. 'F' stands for 'fourth', similar to the quartile which cuts off 25% of a distribution, next to the letter is the depth of the fourth, 6.5, denoting that the lower fourth is the average of the sixth lowest observation with the next above it and the upper fourth is the average of the sixth highest observation with the one below it. The fourths themselves are placed side by side in the box. Below them are the extreme values.

Stem-and-leaf and letter-value displays together convey a good deal of information about the set of observations. Neatly done, the stem-and-leaf is sufficiently graph-like that one can appreciate the shape of the distribution of the observations. Attention is drawn to any unusual values which can then be checked to see whether they are real or whether they have arisen from a copying error. The median summarizes the location of the observations and it is resistant, that is, insensitive to the influence of a few unusual values in the set of observations. The dispersion of the observations is indicated by the fourth-spread, or F-spread, the difference between the upper fourth and the lower fourth; a measure of dispersion which is both simple and also resistant.

The resistance of the F-spread to outlying values can be used to identify 'outside values' for special examination. A practical rule[2] is to cut off any observations which lie outside the limits of 1.5 F-spreads above and below the fourths, designating these as 'outside values'[3]. Less than 1% of a normal distribution would be outside, but small samples from a normal distribution are less well behaved - about 2.4% of observations in samples of size 24 would be outside values. Thus in the example of Table 5.2 and Figure 5.1 there are no outside values and this is consistent with a dispersion similar to that in a sample from a normal distribution.

BOX PLOTS

The outside cut-offs can be combined graphically with the information in the letter-display to show much of the structure of the set of observations (Figure 5.2). The median is shown by the crossbar inside the box; it summarizes the location of the observations. The F-spread is represented by the length of the box, showing the dispersion of the observations. The most extreme observations of Table 5.2 fall well within the outside cut-offs, both upper and lower, therefore the cut-offs are not shown in Figure 5.2. In this case the whiskers are drawn extending only as far as the extreme upper and lower observations, but when there are outside values, the whiskers terminate at the cut-off points 1.5 F-spreads from the ends of the box, and the outside values are shown as points (possibly labelled as well). In Figure 5.2, the positions of the median and lower fourth, closer together than to the upper fourth, show at once that the observations are slightly skewed. The box plot is a visual summary particularly valuable for showing how a set of observations is different from a normally distributed set[4]. The example is of a slightly skewed set with dispersion no greater than would be expected if it was drawn from a normal distribution.

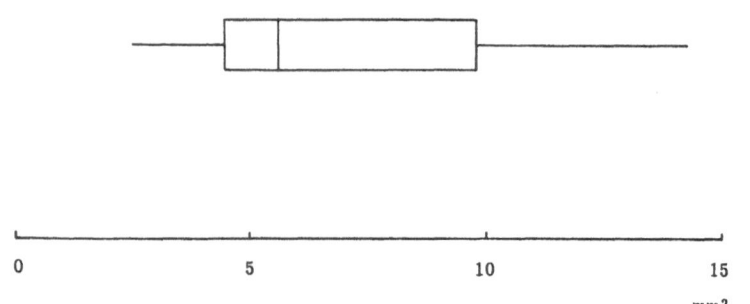

Figure 5.2 Box plots of observations from Table 5.2 and Figure 5.1 showing minimum and maximum values, median and F-spread

CONCLUSION

Measurements of physical properties of the skin need appropriate summaries. The choice is likely to be better directed if the collected observations have been examined and explored using some graphical technique and thus making use of the natural expertise of the eye and brain in pattern recognition. The stem-and-leaf display and its developement, the box plot, are practical and quick methods which help us to understand our observations and make sense of the numbers we have collected.

ACKNOWLEDGEMENTS

I wish to acknowledge the generosity of my colleagues, Dr K Dalziel and Dr M Takahashi, who allowed me to use some of their data for my examples.

REFERENCES

1. Cox, D.R. and Snell, E.J. (1981). Applied Statistics: Principles and Examples. (London: Chapman & Hall)
2. Tukey, J.W. (1977). Exploratory Data Analysis. (Massachusetts: Addison-Wesley)
3. Hoaglin, D., Mosteller, F. and Tukey, J.W. (1983). Understanding Robust and Exploratory Data Analysis. (New York: John Wiley & Sons)
4. Hartwig, F. and Dearing, B.E. (1979). Exploratory Data Analysis. (Beverly Hills: Sage Publications)

Section II

BARRIER PROPERTIES
OF THE SKIN

Chapter 6

The skin as an
immunological barrier

S M Breathnach

INTRODUCTION

The skin is the largest organ in the body, and acts as the principal interface with the external environment; as such, it is often the first organ to come into contact with harmful allergens. It is therefore not too surprising to find that advances in the past decade have demonstrated that normal mammalian epidermis functions as an immunological organ, consisting of resident bone marrow-derived, dendritic antigen-presenting Langerhans cells (LC), and keratinocytes which secrete a variety of immunoregulatory cytokines[1-4]. It has been postulated that normal individuals possess subpopulations of T cells which preferentially home to, and recirculate through, the skin; neoplastic T helper cells which infiltrate the epidermis in lesions of cutaneous T cell lymphoma may represent the malignant counterpart of such epidermotropic T cells[5,6]. It has accordingly been proposed that LC, keratinocytes, epidermotropic T cells and draining peripheral lymph nodes collectively form an integrated system of 'skin-associated lymphoid tissues (SALT)' which mediates cutaneous immunosurveillance[7].

LANGERHANS CELLS

Suprabasal dendritic cells within the epidermis which stain with the Cohnheim gold chloride technique were first described by Paul Langerhans in 1868. LC, which constitute about 2% of epidermal cells, are identified ultrastructurally by the presence of a characteristic cytoplasmic granule[8]; cells which resemble LC ultrastructurally, but lack the characteristic granule, are termed indeterminate cells. Studies with chimeras have revealed that LC are derived from the bone marrow[1]. LC express membrane ATPase and a number of macrophage-type surface markers including FcIgG and C3 receptors[1-3]. LC in human epidermis also express T6/Leu 6 antigen[9]. LC and indeterminate cells are the only cells in normal epidermis which express Ia/HLA-DR (immune response-associated) antigen[1-3]. LC are capable of performing the same antigen-presenting function in the epidermis as Ia$^+$ macrophages do in other body organs. LC provide both signals necessary for T helper cell activation, in that they take up and process antigen and present it in the context of histocompatible Ia antigen, and they also secrete the cytokine interleukin 1 (IL-1)[10-15]. IL-1 triggers production of interleukin 2 (IL-2, T cell growth factor) by helper T cells, which in turn promotes T cell proliferation and differentiation. The antigen-presenting capacity of LC has been demonstrated chiefly by the in vitro mixed epidermal cell-lymphocyte reaction, in which LC induce allogeneic and antigen-specific T cell activation and generation of cytotoxic T cells[10-14].

KERATINOCYTE-DERIVED CYTOKINES

Epidermal cell-derived thymocyte activating factor (ETAF) is a polypeptide of molecular weight approximately 15 kd, which is spontaneously secreted by keratinocytes in vitro, and is produced in greater quantities in response to various noxious stimuli[4,16,17]. ETAF, which is indistinguishable from IL-1[4,17], is chemotactic for polymorphonuclear, mononuclear and T cells[18,19], stimulates fibroblast proliferation and collagenase and prostaglandin production, and induces fever and an acute phase response following parenteral injection in animals[4]. ETAF has been proposed as a mediator of cutaneous inflammation in view of its immunoregulatory function, and its IL-2 enhancing and chemotactic properties[4,20]. Keratinocytes spontaneously secrete a variety of other immunoregulatory cytokines including a cytokine which is indistinguishable from lymphocyte-derived interleukin 3[21], which promotes the growth of cells of haematopoietic lineage and induces mast cell activation and proliferation, and a cytokine which augments natural killer cell activity[22]. Keratinocytes have also been reported to secrete prostaglandin E_2, leukotrienes and interferon.

EPIDERMOTROPIC T LYMPHOCYTES

Central to our present concept of the skin as an organ responsible for immunosurveillance against noxious allergens in the external environment, as embodied in the SALT hypothesis, is the tenet that epidermotropic T cells constantly travel through and sample the epidermis on their path from the circulation to the regional lymph nodes and back. The recent identification of a subset of dendritic Thy-1 antigen-bearing, bone marrow-derived epidermal cells, distinct from but present in equivalent numbers to LC, in murine epidermis[23-25] has excited considerable interest, since Thy-1 antigen in the mouse is especially a marker for peripheral T lymphocytes. It has therefore been proposed that these Thy-1$^+$ dendritic epidermal cells might represent epidermotropic T cells[24]. However, Thy-1$^+$ dendritic epidermal cells do not express the conventional murine T cell markers Lyt 1, 2 or 3, and although they express the natural killer cell marker asialo GM_1[26], we have been unable to demonstrate any natural killer cell function of these cells (Breathnach, Caughman and Katz, unpublished).

We sought to identify a potential human analogue of the murine Thy-1$^+$ dendritic epidermal cell utilizing a battery of antileukocyte reagents in immunohistochemical, flow cytometric and cell sorting studies[27]. Immunofluorescence staining with both anti-murine and anti-human Thy-1 antibodies failed to demonstrate a population of Thy-1[+] cells in human epidermis. Thy-1 antigen in the human, unlike the mouse, is not present on peripheral blood leukocytes; therefore negative staining with anti-Thy-1 antibody alone does not exclude the possible existence of a human analogue. However, a panel of antibodies including anti-asialo GM_1 failed to detect significant numbers of T cells, B cells, monocytes/macrophages other than LC, or natural killer cells in tissue sections, epidermal sheets, or epidermal cell suspensions enriched for leukocyte subpopulations by Ficoll-Hypaque density gradient centrifugation. It is accordingly unlikely that an analogue of the murine Thy-1[+] dendritic epidermal cell exists in human epidermis. In addition, the mean number of cells expressing T cell markers in the epidermis as assessed by fluorescence microscopy of epidermal sheets was only 0.25 per mm^2, compared with 608 LC per mm^2. T cells constituted only 0.16% of all epidermal cells in suspension, even when the suspensions were substantially enriched for mononuclear cell subpopulations by density gradient centrifugation, as determined by flow cytometric analysis. These findings call into question the occurrence of a significant degree of T cell epidermotropism in normal adult human skin. This does not, of course, exclude an important role for epidermotropic T cells in conditions, such as allergic contact dermatitis, involving epidermal inflammation.

ALLERGIC CONTACT DERMATITIS

Analysis of the sequence of events which occurs following epicutaneous applications of allergen, in the induction and elicitation phases of allergic contact dermatitis, provides a very useful model for our understanding of how the various elements of the skin-associated lymphoid tissues interact in order to ensure an integrated response to cutaneous neoantigens. By virtue of their antigen presenting capacity, Ia[+]/HLA-DR[+] LC are thought to play a critical role in the development of allergic contact dermatitis[1-3]. The number of epidermal HLA-DR[+],T6[+] LC is increased in the early stages (12 hours) of allergic contact dermatitis and delayed type hypersensitivity reactions[28-30]. Epicutaneously applied allergen associates with keratinocytes and epidermal LC within 1 hour, and appears in association with upper dermal dendritic cells within 6 hours[28]. HLA-DR[+],T6[+] LC appear in increased numbers in the upper dermis from 6 hours onwards[28,29,31-33]. Electron microscopy has revealed close apposition between infiltrating mononuclear cells and LC in the epidermis and dermis[28,31,34]. LC have been observed in dermal vessels resembling lymphatics after challenge with contact allergens, and in draining lymph nodes following intradermal challenge in sensitized animals[35]. These findings have led to the concept that antigen-bearing LC migrate to draining lymph nodes, and may present antigen to lymphocytes in the epidermis, dermis or in the lymph nodes.

Although keratinocytes do not generally express Ia/HLA-DR antigen in normal skin, they have been reported to express Ia/HLA-DR antigen in a variety of lymphocyte-mediated skin diseases, including allergic contact dermatitis, the tuberculin reaction, lichen planus, mycosis fungoides/cutaneous T cell lymphoma, lupus erythematosus, allograft rejection, and cutaneous graft-versus-host disease[36]. Expression of Ia/HLA-DR antigen by other normally Ia/HLA-DR negative cell types, including thyroid epithelial cells in autoimmune thyroiditis, has resulted in the cells developing the capacity to present antigen. It has therefore been suggested that ETAF/IL-1-secreting keratinocytes which acquire surface Ia/HLA-DR may be able to present antigen directly to T lymphocytes, thereby greatly enhancing the cutaneous immune response to neoantigens[36].

Antigen presentation by LC to T helper cells in the skin or in the regional lymph nodes results in the generation of primed antigen-specific T cells, which mediate the delayed-type hypersensitivity and cytotoxic reactions of allergic contact dermatitis. Following re-presentation of the contact allergen by LC in the epidermis or the dermis in a challenge reaction, such primed antigen-specific effector T cells release lymphokines, resulting in the upper dermal perivascular lymphocytic infiltration, lymphocyte exocytosis and epidermal spongiosis typical of the histology of acute allergic contact dermatitis. Although mechanisms exist for the preferential recruitment of antigen-specific T cells from the circulation to sites of challenge with specific contact allergens, the great majority of cells in the dermal inflammatory infiltrate will have been recruited non-specifically[37]. Indeed, several studies have shown no significant difference in the kinetics and cellular composition of such dermal infiltrates between allergic and irritant contact dermatitis reactions[32,38] (see also Chapter 9). Nevertheless, small numbers of antigen-specific T cells may be retained in previous sites of contact sensitivity for prolonged periods, resulting in local specific immunological memory which may be important in retest or flare-up reactivity[39].

Epicutaneous applications of allergen results not only in the generation of antigen-specific effector T cells, but also of antigen-specific suppressor cells which down-regulate and modulate the immunological response under conditions of normal immunization[37]. The degree of immunity achieved therefore reflects a balance between active sensitization and specific tolerance; whether the balance shifts in favour of immunity or suppression may be a function of the nature and dose of the allergen, of whether there has been prior exposure to the allergen by a parenteral route, and of the susceptibility to contact sensitization of the individual concerned. In addition to antigen-specific suppressor T cells, the modulation of contact sensitivity reactions involves contrasuppressor T cells which prevent suppressor T cells from inhibiting helper T cells, and suppressor B cells, which secrete auto-anti-receptor antibodies[37].

CONCLUSION

The immunological response to an allergen applied to the skin involves interaction between antigen presenting epidermal LC, cytokine-secreting keratinocytes, and T cells of various functional types. Thus the skin, and in particular the epidermis, functions as the most peripheral outpost of the body's immune system, and participates in the formation of an 'immunological barrier' for the detection of noxious exogenous or neoantigens at the skin surface.

REFERENCES

1. Stingl, G., Tamaki, K. and Katz, S.I. (1980). Origin and function of epidermal Langerhans cells. Immunol. Rev., **53**, 149-74
2. Rowden, G. (1981). The Langerhans cell. CRC Crit. Rev. Immunol., **3**, 94-180
3. Wolff, K. and Stingl, G. (1983). The Langerhans cell. J. Invest. Dermatol., **80** (suppl 6), 17-21s
4. Luger, T.A., Kock, A., Danner, M., Colot, M. and Micksche, M. (1985). Production of distinct cytokines by epidermal cells. Br. J. Dermatol., **113**, (suppl 28), 145-56
5. Patterson, J.A.F. and Edelson, R.L. (1978). Interaction of T cells with the epidermis. Br. J. Dermatol., **107**, 117-22
6. Streilein, J.W. (1978). Lymphocyte traffic, T cell malignancies and the skin. J. Invest. Dermatol., **71**, 167-71
7. Streilein, J.W. (1983). Skin-associated lymphoid tissues (SALT): origins and functions. J. Invest. Dermatol., **80** (suppl 6), 12-16s
8. Birbeck, M.S., Breathnach, A.S. and Everall, J.D. (1961). An electron microscopic study of basal melanocytes and high level clear cells (Langerhans cell) in vitiligo. J. Invest. Dermatol., **37**, 51-64
9. Fithian, E., Kung, P., Goldstein, G., Rubenfield, M., Fenoglio, C. and Edelson, R. (1981). Reactivity of Langerhans cells with hybridoma antibody. Proc. Natl. Acad. Sci. USA, **78**, 2541-4
10. Stingl, G., Katz, S.I., Clement, L., Green, I. and Shevach, E.M. (1978). Immunologic functions of Ia-bearing epidermal Langerhans cells. J. Immunol., **121**, 2005-13
11. Braathen, L.R. and Thorsby, E. (1980). Studies on human epidermal Langerhans cells. Allo-activating and antigen-presenting capacity. Scand. J. Immunol., **11**, 401-8
12. Czernielewski, J., Schmitt, D., Faure, M. and Thivolet, J. (1983). Functional and phenotypic analysis of isolated human Langerhans cells and indeterminate cells. Br. J. Dermatol., **108**, 129-38
13. Pehamberger, H., Stingl, L.A., Pogantsch, S., Steiner, G., Wolff, K. and Stingl, G. (1983). Epidermal cell-induced generation of cytotoxic T lymphocytes against alloantigens or TNP-modified syngeneic cells: requirement for Ia-positive Langerhans cells. J. Invest. Dermatol., **81**, 208-11
14. Faure, M., Frappaz, A., Schmitt, D., Dezutter-Dambuyant, C. and Thivolet, J. (1984). Role of HLA-DR bearing Langerhans cells and epidermal indeterminate cells in the in vitro generation of alloreactive cytotoxic T cells in man. Cell. Immunol., **83**, 271-9
15. Sauder, D.N., Dinarello, C.A. and Morhenn, V.B. (1984). Langerhans cell production of interleukin-1. J. Invest. Dermatol., **82**, 605-7
16. Sauder, D.N., Carter, C.S., Katz, S.I. and Oppenheim, J.J. (1982). Epidermal cell production of thymocyte activating factor (ETAF). J. Invest. Dermatol., **79**, 34-9
17. Luger, T.A., Stadler, B.M., Luger, B.M., Mathieson, B.J., Mage, M., Schmidt, J.A. and Oppenheim, J.J. (1982). Murine epidermal cell-derived thymocyte-activating factor resembles murine interleukin 1. J. Immunol., **128**, 2147-52
18. Luger, T.A., Charon, J.A., Colot, M., Micksche, M. and Oppenheim, J.J. (1983). Chemotactic properties of partially purified human epidermal cell-derived thymocyte-activating factor (ETAF) for polymorphonuclear and mononuclear cells. J. Immunol., **131**, 816-20
19. Sauder, D.N., Monick, M. and Hunninghake, G. (1984). Human epidermal cell derived thymocyte activating factor is a potent T cell chemoattractant (abstract). Clin. Res., **32**, 613A
20. Sauder, D.N. and Katz, S.I. (1982). Immune modulation by epidermal cell products: possible role of ETAF in inflammatory and neoplastic skin diseases. J. Am. Acad. Dermatol., **7**, 651-4

21. Luger, T.A., Wirth, U. and Kock, A. (1985). Epidermal cells synthesize a cytokine with interleukin 3-like properties. J. Immunol., **134**, 915-9

22. Luger, T.A., Uchida, A., Kock, A., Colot, M. and Micksche, M. (1985). Human epidermal cells and squamous carcinoma cells synthesize a cytokine that augments natural killer cell activity. J. Immunol., **134**, 2477-83

23. Tschachler, E., Schuler, G., Hutterer, J., Leibl, H., Wolff, K. and Stingl, G. (1983). Expression of Thy-1 antigen by murine epidermal cells. J. Invest. Dermatol., **81**, 282-5

24. Bergstresser, P.R., Tigelaar, R.E., Dees, J.H. and Streilein, J.W. (1983). Thy-1 antigen-bearing dendritic cells populate murine epidermis. J. Invest. Dermatol., **81**, 286-8

25. Breathnach, S.M. and Katz, S.I. (1984). Thy-1$^+$ dendritic cells in murine epidermis are bone marrow-derived. J. Invest. Dermatol., **83**, 74-7

26. Romani, N., Stingl, G., Tschachler, E., Witmer, M.D., Steinman, R.M., Shevach, E.M. and Schuler, G. (1985). The Thy-1-bearing cell of murine epidermis: a distinctive leukocyte perhaps related to natural killer cells. J. Exp. Med., **161**, 1368-83

27. Cooper, K.D., Breathnach, S.M., Caughman, S.W., Palini, A.G., Waxdal, M.J. and Katz, S.I. (1985). Fluorescence microscopic and flow cytometric analysis of bone marrow-derived cells in human epidermis: a search for the human analogue of the murine dendritic Thy-1$^+$ epidermal cell. J. Invest. Dermatol., **85**, 546-52

28. Carr, M.M., Botham, P.A., Gawrodger, D.J., Mcvittie, E., Ross, J.A., Stewart, I.C. and Hunter, J.A.A. (1984). Early cellular reactions induced by dinitrochlorobenzene in sensitized human skin. Br. J. Dermatol., **110**, 637-41

29. Poulter, L.W., Seymour, G.J., Duke, O., Janossy, G. and Panayi, G. (1982). Immunohistological analysis of delayed-type hypersensitivity in man. Cell. Immunol., **74**, 358-69

30. MacKie, R.M. and Turbitt, M.L. (1983). Quantitation of dendritic cells in normal and abnormal human epidermis using monoclonal antibodies directed against Ia and HTA antigens. J. Invest. Dermatol., **81**, 216-20

31. Silberberg, I., Baer, R.L. and Rosenthal, S.A. (1976). The role of Langerhans cells in allergic contact hypersensitivity. A review of findings in man and guinea pigs. J. Invest. Dermatol., **66**, 210-17

32. Scheynius, A., Fischer, T., Forsum, U. and Klareskog, L. (1984). Phenotype characterization in situ of inflammatory cells in allergic and irritant contact dermatitis in man. Clin. Exp. Immunol., **55**, 81-90

33. Ralfkiaer, E. and Wantzin, G.L. (1984). In situ immunological characterization of the infiltrating cells in positive patch tests. Br. J. Dermatol., **111**, 13-22

34. Silberberg, I. (1973). Apposition of mononuclear cells in Langerhans cells in contact allergic reactions. An ultrastructural study. Acta Dermatovener. (Stockh.), **53**, 1-12

35. Silberberg-Sinakin, I., Thorbecke, G.J., Baer, R.L., Rosenthal, S.A. and Berezowsky, V. (1976). Antigen-bearing Langerhans cells in skin, dermal lymphatics and in lymph nodes. Cell. Immunol., **25**, 137-51

36. Breathnach, S.M. and Katz, S.I. (1986). Cell mediated immunity and the skin. Hum. Pathol., **17**, 161-7

37. Breathnach, S.M. (1986). Immunological aspects of contact dermatitis. In Guin, J. and Beaman, J. (eds.) Plant Dermatitis. Clinics in Dermatology (Philadelphia: J.B. Lippincott) **4** (2), 5-17

38. Kanerva, L., Ranki, A. and Lauharanta, J. (1984). Lymphocytes and Langerhans cells in patch tests. An immunohistochemical and electron microscopic study. Contact Dermatol., **11**, 150-5

39. Scheper, R.J., von Blomberg, M., Boerrigter, G.H., Bruynzeel, D., van Dinther, A. and Vos, A. (1983). Induction of immunological memory in the skin. Role of local T cell retention. Clin. Exp. Immunol., **51**, 141-8

Chapter 7

The skin as a microbial barrier

C M Philpot

INTRODUCTION

The skin is a tough, resistant, multi-layered structure of the exterior of the body, whose main function is protective. The outermost layer, the stratum corneum, is the main barrier to microbial invasion, but the inner living layers also have a role, particularly in combating infection[1].

Certain conditions are important in maintaining the barrier function. They also influence the growth of microorganisms on the skin, and thus the role these organisms play in the development of infection. These conditions are:

(1) pH: usually acid (although a neutral-alkaline pH is recorded in occluded areas, e.g. axillae, anogenital areas), due to lactic acid and other acids in sweat and epidermal tissues.

(2) Humidity: 90-100% depending upon site.

(3) CO_2-O_2 balance: little is known about the effect of this on the microbial flora or in pathogenesis of infection. Reduced O_2 or increased CO_2 is thought to be one of the factors encouraging the development of ringworm[2], and affects the growth of microaerophilic organisms, e.g. P. acnes.

(4) Temperature: multiplication of bacteria and fungi increases as the temperature rises; some infections are more common in temperate climates than in tropical countries. The presence of a large inoculum, i.e. microorganisms, is one of the important factors in establishing experimental infections.

The stratum corneum is covered with a film made up of the products of keratinization (desquamated corneocytes), sweat and products of sebaceous glands (surface lipids), and a unique microbial flora, whose relative composition varies from site to site. These also vary with age, sex, site, diet, disease, etc.

Eccrine sweat is composed largely of water, with various trace elements, organic substances and amino acids[3] but it lacks lipids. Alterations in trace substances have been recorded in certain disease states, e.g. psoriasis, ringworm. Some of these trace substances are utilized by the skin flora and this may be of importance in the distribution among different sites and micro-environments. The same substances in higher concentrations may

61

also be inhibitory. Much of the work has been carried out in vitro and the findings extrapolated to the situation in vivo. Immunoglobulins have also been detected in sweat, and increases in some reported, e.g. IgE in atopics and similar, but very little information is available[3].

Sebum is composed of triglycerides, esters, cholesterol and squalene, which make up the skin surface lipids. There has been much argument about the role of sebum, ranging from Kligman[4] who maintained that its only function was to prevent desiccation, to those who believe it plays an active role in preventing the multiplication of pathogenic organisms[5]. Removal of lipids by organic solvents reduces the water holding capacity of the epidermis, but there is little evidence that this occurs under natural conditions[3].

The presence of skin lipids is important for the survival of bacteria on the skin. Removal or binding of lipids enhances the survival of Staphylococcus aureus and Streptococci, although Gram negative bacteria are less affected[3]. Pityrosporum orbiculare and Pr. acnes are stimulated by long chain fatty acids, and are found particularly in areas with high levels of these substances.

Many bacteria and fungi[6,7] produce lipases in vitro that split triglycerides; however, it is less certain that these are effective in vivo.

THE NORMAL FLORA

The normal flora consists essentially of aerobic cocci and diphtheroids, both on dry skin and in wetter areas. In addition there are microaerophilic, lipid-loving corynebacteria and yeasts on forehead, scalp and other lipid rich areas. The role of the resident microflora in the prevention of infection has been investigated with some thoroughness and appears primarily to be the prevention of the multiplication of pathogenic organisms. It also competes for binding sites on epidermal cells. Application of antibiotics, disinfectants or occlusive dressings may alter the normal flora which then may be replaced by other, potentially pathogenic, organisms. This may also occur in disease states such as eczema in which S. aureus may colonize the skin. Some organisms, e.g. Pr. acnes and P. orbiculare, may, under conditions not always well defined, become pathogenic themselves.

FACTORS PREDISPOSING TO INFECTION

The stratum corneum provides a very satisfactory barrier to microbial penetration under normal circumstances, but this function may be lost if its nature is altered in any way. There are several ways in which this alteration may be achieved.

Desiccation

When water loss from epidermal cells exceeds intake, or the relative humidity drops as in cold or windy weather, the stratum corneum can dry and crack, thus allowing the entry of microbes, e.g. in infective eczema.

Physical trauma

Removing part or all of the stratum corneum by scratching or maceration allows microbes to enter. From experimental infections, it appears that streptococci can only invade if there is an actual break in the skin[8]; they do not survive long on intact skin particularly if it is dry although 'skin' strains last longer. Staphylococci are also invasive when the skin has been subjected to trauma, but other factors are probably more important[3]. It was established by Knight[9] and other workers[10] that trauma to the skin actually had an adverse effect on the survival of ringworm fungi if it was too severe, due to the leakage of 'serum' into the stratum corneum and its inhibition of fungal growth.

Hydration

This appears to be a most important factor in the establishment of bacterial and fungal infections. Increased water alters the corneocytes, so that their barrier efficiency is decreased[1]. This has been demonstrated both in experimental and in natural infections. The virulent nature of the bacterial and fungal infections in the combat soldiers in Vietnam was ascribed to the fact that their skin was kept continuously sodden[11,12]. Other workers have reported greatly increased rates of infection in tropical countries, particularly infections in sites kept warm and moist by various means[12,13], e.g. occlusion (dressings, ointments, clothes). It has been suggested that the presence of water on skin allows microbial antibiotics to diffuse more freely[3].

The establishment of microbial skin disease, as opposed to mere colonization of the skin, reflects the interplay of a number of factors:

(1) hydration (high humidity);
(2) the presence of a large inoculum;
(3) the 'virulence' of the infecting pathogen (e.g special phage types of S. aureus);
(4) trauma to the stratum corneum;
(5) the presence of other diseases;
(6) the age of the patient;
(7) the rate at which desquamation of epithelial cells removes microorganisms;

(8) the carriage (especially the continuous carriage) of staphylococci and streptococci.

From the difficulty of establishing experimental infections with either bacteria or fungi, without the use of chemical or mechanical damage to the stratum corneum, the prime factor would undoubtedly appear to be the alteration of this protective layer.

'SUBCORNEAL' HOST RESISTANCE

Once the stratum corneum has been breached other factors come into play. Bacterial toxins and enzymes can attack both cells and intercellular material of the epidermis. Ringworm fungi produce proteases in vitro; it seems certain that in vivo they hydrolyse the intercellular materials and produce keratinases that can attack keratin or perhaps keratin altered in some manner[14,15]. After a variable period of time, the clinical lesion appears. The way in which the host resists and combats infection involves a variety of factors in both epidermis and dermis. This may be illustrated by fungal infection. The development of the clinical lesion is followed, immunologically, by the development of delayed type hypersensitivity to the fungus as shown by the trichophytin test[16], and histopathologically by hyphae becoming surrounded by polymorphonuclear leukocytes; there is a great increase in the thickness of the stratum corneum. The enclosed mycelial mass eventually separates from the epidermis, a crust is formed and the whole is sloughed off[17,18]. If a second infection is induced at the same or nearby site, a similar sequence of events occurs, but much more rapidly.

THE EFFECTS OF DESQUAMATION

The rate of epidermal turnover of cells is normally sufficient to replace the stratum corneum without increasing or decreasing the thickness. Scaling and thickening are features of many skin diseases, e.g. psoriasis, eczema. The balance is between proliferation of the organism and the rate at which the stratum corneum is renewed, so if the pathogen multiplies faster, the lesion spreads, and if the turnover increases faster, the pathogen is shed. In experimental lesions with Candida albicans, Sohnle and co-workers[19,20] showed that there must have been an increased turnover of epidermal cells in the lesion since large numbers of basal cells were labelled with tritiated thymidine, indicating active mitosis. Tosti and co-workers[21] found in pityriasis versicolor that the yeasts were carried up with epidermal scales, but mycelium grew downwards, and persistence of the lesion was determined by a dynamic balance between growth and multiplication of organisms and rate of renewal of the horny layer. It has been suggested that psoriatics do not get ringworm because of the increased epidermal turnover in psoriatic lesions, although ringworm infections have been induced experimentally and also found clinically. Berk and co-workers[22], with the same technique, found an increased epidermal turnover at the edge but not in the centre of the lesions. They suggested that the increased turnover at the rim of the lesion was a direct response of the epidermis to the presence of the fungus causing shedding of the fungus, repair of the damage and also modification of the cells to make them unsuitable for fungal growth. The fungus continued to grow outwards stimulating further reaction at the edge of the lesion while in the centre, host defence substances (unspecified) might be inactivating the fungus.

SERUM FACTORS

The restriction of ringworm fungi and yeasts to the stratum corneum except under certain well-defined and very rare conditions, suggests that host factors must be important. It was early established that serum derived from patients[23,24] was inhibitory to the growth of the fungi. This factor or factors did not appear to be related to the 'id' reaction or hypersensitivity to trichophytin[25]. Absence of this factor permitted the fungi to invade beyond the stratum corneum[26]. This factor was identified as unsaturated transferrin by King and co-workers[27], and it was suggested that transferrin in serum diffused through the epidermis to the stratum corneum and inhibited fungal growth[16], although there is little real evidence for this.

Other 'serum factors' have been described, which possibly inhibit the fungal proteolytic enzymes. Normal serum inhibits the proteolytic keratinase of T. mentagrophytes, and the inhibitor has been isolated and identified as α-2-macroglobulin[28].

It has been suggested that the inflammation associated with clinical lesions results in greater exudation of serum and thus increased inhibition of fungi in the skin[9].

CELL-MEDIATED IMMUNITY

Sohnle and Kirkpatrick[20] showed that the presence of cell-mediated immunity influenced the rate at which desquamation occurred. Animals that were immunized prior to infection showed a greater rate of labelling of basal cells, a far more marked scaling response, and greatly increased acanthosis, parakeratosis and hyperkeratosis of the epidermis, compared to non-immunized animals. They suggested that cell-mediated immunity affects the mitotic rate, and thus the rate at which skin cells are shed. They also noted that the onset of cellular immunity and the increased rate of desquamation were much more rapid in those lesions that were occuluded[19].

The production of humoral antibody is important in the development of resistance to invasion by staphylococci and streptococci. In fungal infections, the onset of inflammation and the resolution of the lesion coincide with the development of delayed-type cutaneous hypersensitivity particularly to the polysaccharide components of the fungi[15]. The importance of cell-mediated (T cell) response to invasion in the resolution of infection is underlined by the lack of response in those individuals who develop spreading or chronic infections. Their lymphocytes lack the ability to respond specifically to fungal infections[29]. There are various theories to explain this lack of reactivity on the part of the skin: blocking of the delayed-type hypersensitivity by Type 1 reactivity and circulating antibodies (often found in chronic infections - there is a significant correlation between the presence of atopy and the development of chronic infection); local trapping of lymphocytes so that they fail to respond; epidermal cell binding of antigen; overproduction of antigen so that a state of cellular tolerance is achieved; or T cell reactivity may be blocked by suppressor T or B cells[16]. Kaaman and co-workers have reported finding a decreased proportion of T helper cells and increased numbers of T suppressor cells in patients with chronic infections[30].

It is not yet certain how antigen in the stratum corneum comes into contact with immunocompetent cells in the dermis. It has been suggested that products of inflammation such as lymphocytotoxins act directly on host cells and cause damage to the dermal-epidermal barrier. Various workers have demonstrated in vitro that ringworm fungi and yeasts can produce substances chemotactic for polymorphonuclear leukocytes and other cells and can activate complement by the alternate pathway[31-33]. Lymphocytes accumulating in the dermis below the lesion in vitro respond to soluble Candida antigens with the release of lymphokines[19]. These lymphokines may then act on the basal cell layer and induce them to divide more rapidly. The yeasts are not killed by the inflammatory cells, but are removed by the crusting and scaling that accompanies the influx of cells into the epidermis. Tagami showed that chemotactic factors were produced both by the fungus and the lesion, and the lesion extracts also activated complement by the alternate pathway[34]. He suggested that the crusting and scaling were a product of an increased epidermal turnover that was stimulated both by the influx of cells into the epidermis and by the development of delayed-type hypersensitivity. Sohnle et al. were able to transfer the ability to scale from immunized to non-immunized animals by washed peritoneal exudate cells[19].

Holden, Hay and Macdonald[35], using light and electron microscopy and immunoperoxidase staining, showed that the ringworm hyphae in skin sections lay in lacunae whose walls were coated with dermatophyte-derived material. They believed that it was diffusion of these substances across the epidermis that brought them into contact with cells of the immune system.

Some recent work suggests that it is the epidermal Langerhans cells that are responsible for antigen uptake in ringworm infections[36].

CONCLUSION

The response of the skin to invasion is thus a combination of many factors, such as an increase in the rate at which cells (and thus pathogens) are shed; the production of substances that will inhibit the growth of the pathogen in situ, such as the 'serum factor' inhibiting the growth of ringworm fungi; and the development of both humoral and cell-mediated responses to the microbial antigens. The pathogens themselves, by producing toxins and enzymes that attack cells within the epidermis and antigens that provoke the influx of inflammatory cells into dermis and epidermis, play an active role in inducing this response.

REFERENCES

1. Baker, H. (1979). The skin as a barrier. In Rook, A., Wilkinson, O.S. and Ebling, F.J.G. (eds.) Textbook of Dermatology. 3rd edn., pp 289-98. (Oxford: Blackwell)
2. Allen, A.M. and King, R.D. (1978). Occlusion, carbon dioxide and fungal skin infections. Lancet, 1, 360-1
3. Noble, W.C. (1981). Microbiology of Human Skin. (London: Lloyd-Luke (Medical Books) Ltd.)
4. Kligman, A.M. (1963). The uses of sebum. Br. J. Dermatol., 75, 307-19
5. Ebling, F.J. and Rook, A. (1979). The sebaceous gland. In Rook, A., Wilkinson, O.S. and Ebling, F.J.G. (eds.) Textbook of Dermatology. 3rd edn., pp 1691-1731. (Oxford: Blackwell)
6. Hellgren, L. and Vincent, J. (1980). Lipolytic activity of some dermatophytes. J. Med. Microbiol., 13, 155-7
7. Catterall, M.D., Ward, M.E. and Jacobs, P. (1978). A re-appraisal of the role of Pityrosporum orbiculare in Pityriasis versicolor and the significance of extracellular lipase. J. Invest. Dermatol., 71, 398-401
8. Leyden, J.J., Stewart, R. and Kligman, A.A. (1980). Experimental infections with Group A streptococci in humans. J. Invest. Dermatol., 75, 196-201
9. Knight, A.G. (1972). A review of experimental human fungus infections. J. Invest. Dermatol., 59, 354-8
10. Rosenthal, S.A. and Baer, R.L. (1966). Experiments on the biology of fungous infections of the feet. J. Invest. Dermatol., 47, 568-76
11. Allen, A.M. and Taplin, D. (1973). Epidemic Trichophyton mentagrophytes infections in servicemen. Source of infection, role of environment, host factors and susceptibility. J. Am. Med. Assoc., 226, 864-7
12. Sanderson, P.H. and Sloper, J.C. (1953). Skin disease in the British army in S.E. Asia. I. Influence of environment on skin disease. Br. J. Dermatol., 65, 252-64
13. Desai, S.C. (1966). Epidemicity and clinical features of Trichophyton rubrum infections in the tropics. Derm. Int., 5, 222-4
14. Barlow, A.J.E. and English, M.P. (1973). Fungous diseases. In Rook, A. (ed.) Recent Advances in Dermatology. No. 3, pp 33-68. (London: Churchill Livingstone)
15. Grappel, S.F. (1981). Immunology of surface fungi: dermatophytes. In Nahamias, A.J. and O'Reilly, R.J. (eds.) Immunology of Human Infections. Part I: Bacteria, Mycoplasmae, Chlamydiae and Fungi. pp 495-524. (USA: Plenum Medical Book Co.)
16. Jones, H.E., Reinhardt, J.H. and Rinaldi, M.G. (1974). Acquired immunity to dermatophytes. Arch. Dermatol., 109, 840-8
17. Hay, R.J., Calderon, R.A. and Collins, M.J. (1983). Experimental dermatophytosis: the clinical and histopathologic features of a mouse model using Trichophyton quinkeanum (mouse favus). J. Invest. Dermatol., 81, 270-4
18. Greenberg, J.H., King, R.D., Krebs, S. and Field, R. (1976). A quantitative dermatophyte infection model in the guinea pig - a parallel to the quantitated human infection model. J. Invest. Dermatol., 67, 704-8
19. Sohnle, P.G., Frank, M.M. and Kirkpatrick, C.H. (1976). Mechanisms involved in elimination of organisms from experimental cutaneous Candida albicans infections in guinea pigs. J. Immunol., 117, 523-30
20. Sohnle, P.G. and Kirkpatrick, C.H. (1978). Epidermal proliferation in the defence against experimental cutaneous candidiasis. J. Invest. Dermatol., 70, 130-3
21. Tosti, A., Villardita, S. and Fazzini, M.L. (1972). The parasitic colonization of the horny layer in Tinea versicolor. J. Invest. Dermatol., 59, 233-7
22. Berk, S.H., Penneys, N.S. and Weinstein, G.D. (1976). Epidermal activity in annular dermatophytosis. Arch. Dermatol., 112, 485-8

23. Ayers, S. and Anderson, N.P. (1934). Inhibition of fungi in cultures by blood serum from patients with 'phytid' eruptions. Arch. Derm. Syphilol., **29**, 537-47
24. Peck, S.M., Rosenfeld, H. and Glick, A.W. (1940). Fungistatic power of blood serum. Arch. Derm. Syphilol., **42**, 426-37
25. Lorincz, A.L., Priestley, J.O. and Jacobs, P.A. (1958). Evidence for a humoral mechanism which prevents the growth of dermatophytes. J. Invest. Dermatol., **31**, 15-17
26. Blank, H., Sagami, S., Boyd, C. and Roth, F.J. (1959). The pathogenesis of superficial fungus infections on cultured human skin. Arch. Dermatol., **79**, 524-35
27. King, R.D., Khan, H.A., Foye, J.C., Greenberg, J.H. and Jones, H.E. (1975). Transferrin, iron and dermatophytes. 1. Serum dermatophytes inhibitory component definitively identified as unsaturated transferrin. J. Lab. Clin. Med., **86**, 204-12
28. Yu, R.J., Grappel, S.F. and Blank, F. (1972). Inhibition of keratinases by α2-macroglobulin. Experentia, **28**, 886
29. Ahmed, A.R. (1982). Immunology of human dermatophyte infections. Arch. Dermatol., **118**, 521-5
30. Kaaman, T., Petrini, B. and Wasserman, J. (1983). Immune responses in chronic dermatophytosis. Br. J. Dermatol., **108**, 124-5
31. Davies, R.R. and Zaini, F. (1984). Trichophyton rubrum and the chemotaxis of polymorphonuclear leucocytes. Sabouraudia, **22**, 65-71
32. Davies, R.R. and Zaini, F. (1984). Enzymic activities of Trichophyton rubrum and the chemotaxis of polymorphonuclear leucocytes. Sabouraudia, J. Med. Vet. Mycol., **22**, 235-41
33. Swan, J.W., Dahl, M.V., Coppo, P.A. and Hammerschmidt, D.E. (1983). Complement activity by Trichophyton rubrum. J. Invest. Dermatol., **80**, 156-8
34. Tagami, H., Natsume, N., Aoshima, T., Inoue, F., Suehisa, S. and Yamada, M. (1982). Analysis of transepidermal leukocyte chemotaxis in experimental dermatophytosis in guinea pigs. Arch. Dermatol. Res., **27**, 205-17
35. Holden, C.A., Hay, R.J. and Macdonald, D.M. (1981). The antigenicity of Trichophyton rubrum: in situ studies by an immunoperoxidase technique in light and electron microscopy. Acta Dermatovener., **61**, 207-11
36. Braathen, L.R. and Kaaman, T. (1983). Human epidermal Langerhans cells induce cellular immune response to trichophytin in dermatophytosis. Br. J. Dermatol., **109**, 295-300

Chapter 8

Do we need an artificial skin?

J C Lawrence

Skin loss may involve part or the whole depth of the skin and the underlying tissues may also be involved. Partial skin loss wounds normally heal within 21 days or less irrespective of any local treatment accorded. Yet it is customary for many such wounds to be dressed and part of the purpose of most wound dressings is to replace some of the protection normally provided by skin[1,2]. Full skin thickness wounds will also heal albeit very slowly; the healed wound almost invariably is scarred; contractures and other deformities of the wound together with surrounding tissues including bone are not uncommon. In addition, the epithelium is frail, readily damaged and hence liable to become malignant. Nowadays it is usual to recommend closing all full thickness wounds greater than 15 cm^2 with autologous skin grafts[3].

Many types of injury can produce partial skin loss wounds, abrasions and many burns afford common examples. Full thickness skin loss is not infrequently a consequence of trauma caused by explosions of all kinds including gun shot; other instances include degloving injuries, amputation and thermal or chemical burns. Similar loss of skin occurs as a consequence of surgery to remove tumours of the skin or breast or if skin blemishes such as port wine stains or tattoos are removed. Infective conditions such as toxic epidermal necrolysis and synergistic gangrenes also cause skin loss.

The use of dressings to treat skin loss is at least as old as recorded history - linen steeped in goat's grease as an application for burns is described in the Ebers papyrus of 1500BC[4] and the practice of treating skin wounds with dressings has continued unabated ever since. Practical readily available wound dressings are scarcely a century old and follow Gamgee's discovery that cotton wool and cotton gauze could be rendered absorbtive by bleaching[5]. Despite a variety of innovative dressings in recent years, some of which are very effective in particular well-defined situations[1,6,7], to date nothing has successfully superseded absorbent cotton for treating areas greater than about 1% of the body surface[8].

It is generally accepted that the most satisfactory closure for defects of the skin is skin, hence the evolution of modern plastic surgery since Reverdin, Thiersch and others first described the successful use of autologous skin grafts about a century ago. Although techniques for resurfacing extensive areas of skin loss are well established sometimes insufficient autologous donor skin is available to close the wound in a single operation. In practical terms the limit is about 10% total body surface area if blood loss and operative time are limited consistent with the well-being of the patient[3]. This area can be increased somewhat by meshing the skin graft which enables it to be expanded. Mesh grafts have disadvantages - the wound is not totally resurfaced immediately and the final cosmetic appearance of the healed wound is less satisfactory than that seen with non-meshed skin. Full skin thickness grafts are also employed to resurface defects over critical areas or when a good cosmetic result is desirable. The problem with such grafts is that the donor area also requires resurfacing though in some instances subcutaneous tissue expanders can be employed thus obviating this secondary problem[9].

With many extensive wounds, complete closure can only be obtained by a series of operations, often over many weeks, relying on donor sites to heal and then be reharvested.

Not surprisingly, application of homologous or heterologous skin has its advocates especially for the treatment of extensive wounds. Skin from a water lizard was used by Canaday in the fifteenth century; more recently homologous skin, usually from close relatives of the patient, has been employed, sometimes as alternate strips with autograft[10]. The ready availability of refrigerators since the Second World war led to the discovery that skin could be stored at 4°C. Epithelial migration from skin so stored can be demonstrated after 21 days or so[11] but viability is not high at this time as measured by skin respiratory activity or succinic dehydrogenase[12]. Two weeks storage may be the upper practical limit if the skin is to take permanently as a graft. However, dead skin may have some merit as a dressing[13].

In recent years liquid nitrogen has become readily available and systems have been designed to store cadaveric and other donor skin at -196°C. Cryoprotective and other manipulative procedures cause some loss of viability[12] but, once stored, there is little further loss of viability over very long periods. Despite sophisticated technology all homologous skin is rejected by the recipient unless the donor happens to be an identical twin. Typical survival time is 2-3 weeks though donor selection by tissue typing can extend this, occasionally by several weeks, but anticipated survival time cannot be accurately predicted. Moreover, if a particular donor is used more than once the second set of grafts are rejected more rapidly than the first[14].

Heterologous skin, usually porcine, is also advocated as a useful means of temporarily closing skin wounds[15]. This is used either fresh or frozen but freeze-dried gamma-irradiated material is possibly the most popular since it is commercially available, readily stored and has a long shelf life. However, it is not antigen free though the dried material appears to be less immunogenic than fresh[15].

Other substitutes for skin have been developed, for example Burke and his colleagues[16] bonded a plastic film to a 'pseudodermis' of collagen plus glycosaminoglycan. **In situ** the 'pseudodermis' becomes permeated by and incorporated within wound granulation tissues; ultimately the outer plastic film is removed and resurfaced with a split thickness skin graft.

It is widely recognized that all of these techniques, whether they be simple application of absorbtive dressings or sophisticated biomaterials, have the fundamental disadvantage that they are only temporary and, although they can reduce some of the problems associated with extensive skin loss such as infection or loss of body fluid, eventually wounds have to be resurfaced with epithelium.

It was therefore logical to turn to tissue culture techniques in an attempt to increase available skin for transplantation. Multiplication of mammalian tissue including skin (but mainly fibroblasts) was achieved many years ago[17] but development of epidermal cell culture has taken much longer. Migration of skin epithelium over the cut surface of split thickness skin explants was described by Medawar[18] in 1948 but this technique does not lend itself to preparing clinically useful skin grafts. More recently Green et al.[19] and O'Connor et al.[20] have devised means of preparing large sheets of epithelial cells from small biopsies of donor skin. The application of this technique together with other 'substitutes' for skin has recently been reviewed by Carney[21]. During the last 18 months the Birmingham Burns Unit has established a laboratory to prepare sheets of cultured epidermal cells to treat extensive burns and results to date are encouraging[22].

Despite the success claimed by several centres for this particular system various aspects need clarification. Billingham and Reynolds[23] found that epidermal grafts did not prevent wound contracture although the cells 'took' satisfactorily. Many authorities argue that epidermis without an underlying dermis will yield an unsatisfactory result; it is not yet clear how valid this criticism is since long-term follow-up including the cosmetic appearance of grafted epidermal sheets has not been reported to date. However, Gallico and O'Connor[24] state that 'further research is necessary so that a skin substitute will truly be a skin replacement'. It seems likely, therefore, that future research will be aimed at producing a graft comprising epidermal cells cultured on sheets of non-immunogenic dermal-like material.

Since the Oxford English Dictionary[25] defines artificial as 'made or produced by art' or 'not natural' it seems that the quest for an artificial skin has been in progress for several thousand years. It is unlikely that generations of clinicians, scientists and philosophers have been searching for a material for which there is no replacement. Moreover, such types of artificial skin that are available are widely used despite their limitations. Fortunately their limitations are recognized and it is likely that considerable development and improvement will follow in the foreseeable future.

REFERENCES

1. Groves, A.R. (1983). Practical aspects of wound dressings. In Lawrence, J.C. (ed.) Wound Healing. pp 115-28. (Oxford: The Medicine Publishing Foundation)
2. Lawrence, J.C. (1982). What materials for dressings? Injury, 13, 500-12
3. Cason, J.S. (1981). Treatment of Burns. (London: Chapman and Hall)
4. Ebell, B. (1937). The Papyrus Ebers. The Greatest Egyptian Medical Document. (Copenhagen: Munksgaard)

5. Gamgee, J.S. (1880). Absorbent and medicated surgical dressings. Lancet, **1**, 127-8
6. Groves, A.R. and Lawrence, J.C. (1985). Silastic foam dressing: an appraisal. Ann. R. Coll. Surg. Engl., **67**, 116-18
7. Groves, A.R. and Lawrence, J.C. (1986). Alginate dressing as a donor site haemostat. Ann. R. Coll. Surg. Engl., **68**, 27-8
8. Groves, A.R. and Lawrence, J.C. (1986). Antibacterial agents and dressings for burns. In Lawrence, J.C. (ed.) Burncare. Hull, Smith and Nephew Medical Ltd.
9. Wyllie, F.J., Gowar, J.P. and Levick, P.L. (1986). Use of tissue expanders after burns and other injuries. Burns, **12**, 277-82
10. Jackson, D.M. (1954). A clinical study of the use of skin homografts for burns. Br. J. Plast. Surg., **7**, 26-42
11. Pepper, F.J. (1954). Studies on the viability of mammalian skin autografts after storage at different temperatures. Br. J. Plast. Surg., **6**, 250-6
12. Lawrence, J.C. (1972). Storage and skin metabolism. Br. J. Plast. Surg., **25**, 440-53
13. Forage, A.V. (1962). The effects of removing the epidermis from burnt skin. Lancet, **2**, 690-3
14. Medawar, P.B. (1944). The behaviour and fate of skin autografts and skin homografts in rabbits. J. Anat., **77**, 299-310
15. Harris, N.S., Compton, J.B., Abston, P. and Larson, D.L. (1976). Comparison of fresh frozen and lyophilised porcine skin as xenografts on burned patients. Burns, **2**, 71-5
16. Burke, J.F., Yannas, I.V., Quimby, W.C., Bondoc, C.C. and Jung, W.K. (1981). Successful use of a physiologically acceptable artificial skin in the treatment of extensive burn injury. Ann. Surg., **194**, 413-28
17. Carell, A. and Burrows, M.T. (1911). Cultivation of tissues in vitro and its technique. J. Exp. Med., **13**, 387-98
18. Medawar, P.B. (1948). The cultivation of adult mammalian skin in vitro. Q. J. Microscop. Sci., **89**, 187-96
19. Green, H., Kehinde, O. and Thomas, J. (1979). Growth of cultured epidermal cells into multiple epithelia suitable for grafting. Proc. Natl. Acad. Sci. USA, **76**, 5665-8
20. O'Connor, N.E., Mulliken, J.B., Banks-Schlegal, S., Kehinde, O. and Green, H. (1981). Grafting of burns with cultured epithelium prepared from autologous epidermal cells. Lancet, **1**, 78-9
21. Carney, S.A. (1986). Generation of autograft; the state of the art. Burns, **12**, 231-5
22. Levick, P. and Blight, A. (1986). The use of epithelial culture in the treatment of burns. Presented at the 19th Annual Meeting of the British Burns Association, Birmingham, April
23. Billingham, R.E.B. and Reynolds, J. (1952). Transplantation studies on sheets of pure epidermal epithelium and on epidermal cell suspensions. Br. J. Plast. Surg., **5**, 25-34
24. Gallico, G.G. and O'Connor, N.E. (1985). Cultured epithelium as a skin substitute. Clin. Plast. Surg., **12**, 149-57
25. Oxford English Dictionary (1985). The Shorter Oxford English Dictionary, 3rd edn. (1944) with subsequent corrections, revisions and addenda. (Oxford: The University Press)

Chapter 9

The skin as a chemical barrier

J D Wilkinson

The skin is an incomplete barrier, water (and some gases) passing through it to some extent. It is also vulnerable to chemical attack.

This barrier property of skin has important therapeutic, toxicological and dermatological consequences[1]. In this paper, I shall concentrate solely on the skin as a chemical barrier in respect to irritants and potential sensitizers.

Cutaneous barrier function resides principally in the stratum corneum, the skin surface lipid film having only a marginal protective effect and also, perhaps, protecting the stratum corneum from microbial attack. There is a second 'theoretical' barrier to cutaneous penetration at the dermo-epidermal interface/basement membrane, although this may simply be no more than a change from a lipophilic to hydrophilic environment resulting in increasing resistance to substances that have previously passed through the predominantly lipophilic stratum corneum with relative ease. Essentially, it is the stratum corneum which provides the principal barrier. Various factors affect this stratum corneum barrier (Table 9.1). Although the stratum corneum varies quite considerably in thickness (e.g between face and palm), an increase in stratum corneum thickness is, to some degree, 'matched' by a decrease in its efficiency, so that the overall barrier function of the skin therefore remains fairly constant.

Table 9.1 Factors affecting skin barrier function

(1) Anatomical

    Stratum corneum thickness/integrity
    'Shunts'
    Stratum corneum reservoir

(2) Biochemical (keratin, lipid, cell wall proteins)

    System of alternating lipophilic and hydrophilic layers

(3) Physiological

    Age, site, presence/absence of skin disease

(4) 'Exogenous'

    Stratum corneum hydration
    Physical trauma
    Chemical trauma
    Temperature

Appendageal 'shunts' are also less important than expected - probably because any chemical entering the follicle or sweat gland apparatus still has to pass through an epithelium before entering the body. Also on the basis of surface area exposed, appendages represent a fairly small portion of the total surface area of the skin. The stratum corneum also acts as a 'reservoir', delaying the entry of noxious chemicals but also, at times, acting as a toxicological store, e.g. hexachlorophane.

The effectiveness of the stratum corneum barrier function varies with site, and to some extent with age, though there is less data on this aspect. The skin of scalp and scrotum is, for example, more permeable than that of the trunk and limbs and these latter sites themselves offer less resistance than the thick skin of palms and soles. Age is not a particularly important factor and only the neonatal or premature infant has significantly impaired skin barrier function. However, the most important 'endogenous' factor as regards stratum corneum barrier function is the presence or absence of skin disease, any disturbance in keratinization resulting in an inefficient barrier.

There are many factors which affect skin barrier function. These include the degree of corneal hydration - both increased hydration and desiccation leading to a loss of barrier function; physical trauma (often underestimated); and chemical trauma, especially the degreasing effect of solvents and detergents. Alternating exposure to solvents and water damages the stratum corneum and allows the leaching out of waterbinding substances. This leads to a rapid deterioration in barrier function.

The skin's resistance to alkali is relatively poor. Also exposure to strong alkali is often initially overlooked since there is often no immediate stinging or burning. Another important factor as regards barrier function is temperature. Irritant reactions are increased both in situations of high temperature and high humidity and also, in the northern hemisphere, during the winter when temperature and relative humidity both fall. This is of practical relevance in respect of the reading of patch test reactions since the intensity of marginally irritant reactions will vary with season.

The skin is also susceptible to the direct effect of irritants. These damage the stratum corneum and, on penetration, the viable epidermis beneath. This often leads to a secondary reduction in barrier function. In general, polar substances penetrate the stratum corneum poorly whereas non-polar (lipid-soluble) and ambiphilic molecules penetrate the stratum corneum with greater ease (Table 9.2). Predicting which chemicals are likely to irritate the skin and which are not is difficult. The response to a substance is often idiosyncratic, highly dependent on its chemical structure and does not appear to be directly related to molecular weight. Individual susceptibility also appears to vary in that the Negro skin appears to be more resistant to both chemical irritation and to induction of allergic contact sensitivity. Patients with eczema, particularly those suffering from seborrhoeic eczema, gravitational eczema or atopic eczema are more easily irritated than those with normal skin.

74

Table 9.2 Penetration of chemicals through the skin

Poor penetration	Easy penetration
Polar	Non-polar (lipid soluble)
Inorganic/organic salts	Substances forming hydrogen bonds, e.g. salicylic acid
Complex polymers	Ambiphilic molecules, e.g. dimethylsulphoxide

The practical expression of these variations in stratum corneum barrier function is reflected in the known propensity of the (occluded) nappy area to irritant reactions and to an increased rate of absorption of applied materials, e.g. topical steroids, hexachlorophane, etc. This may also partly explain the susceptibility of chronically damaged skin sites, such as the lower leg (gravitational eczema) (Figure 9.1) and perineum and ear/eye (sites with chronic or repeated medicament usage), to the development of allergic contact sensitivity. The significance of 'microtrauma' as a cofactor for irritant dermatitis is seen in the palmar and 'extended' finger tip patterns of irritant hand eczema as among housewives, mechanics, etc. (Figure 9.2). The effect of solvents (soaps and detergents) and the loss of water-binding substances from the skin can result in asteatotic eczema (eczema craquelé) (Figure 9.3). In the United Kingdom, both discoid eczema and atopic eczema tend to become worse during the winter months, probably as a result of impaired barrier function and low ambient humidity with subsequent water loss from the skin. Emollients are helpful in all these conditions.

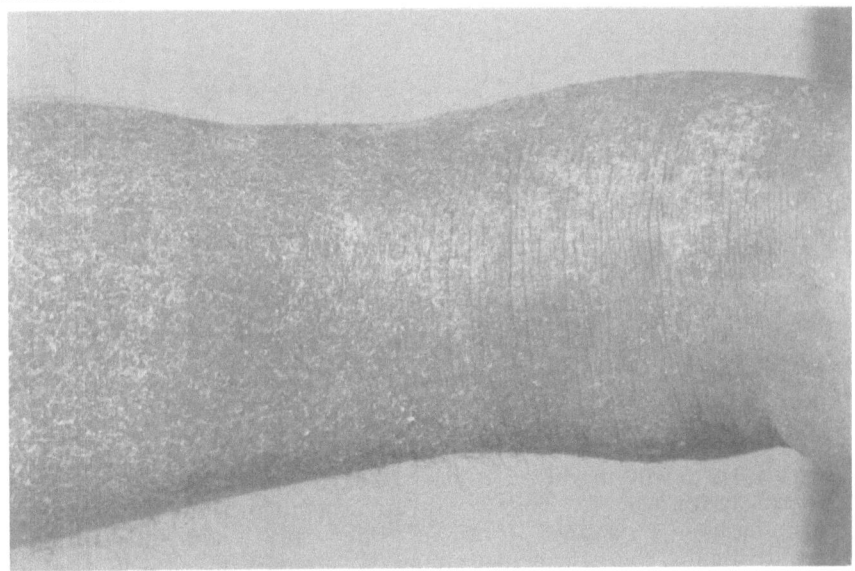

Figure 9.1 Gravitational eczema

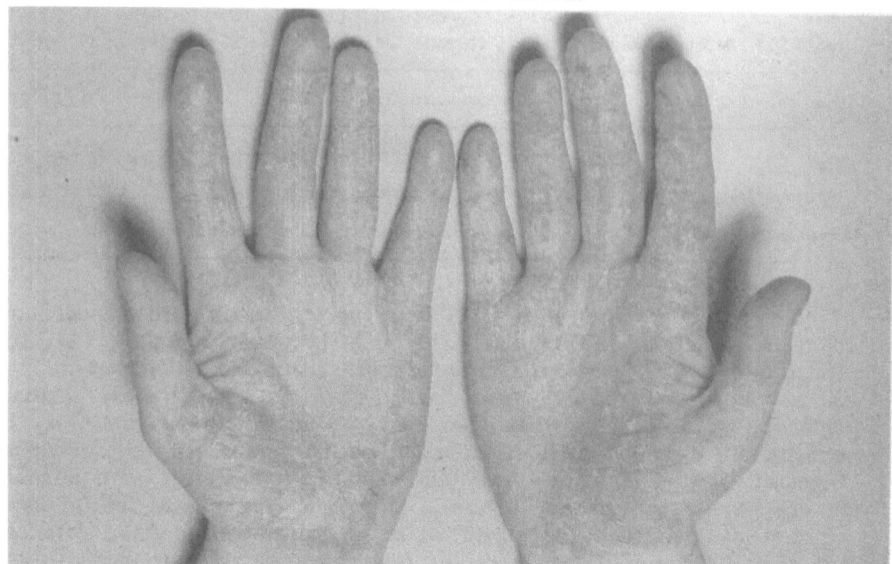

Figure 9.2 Hand eczema

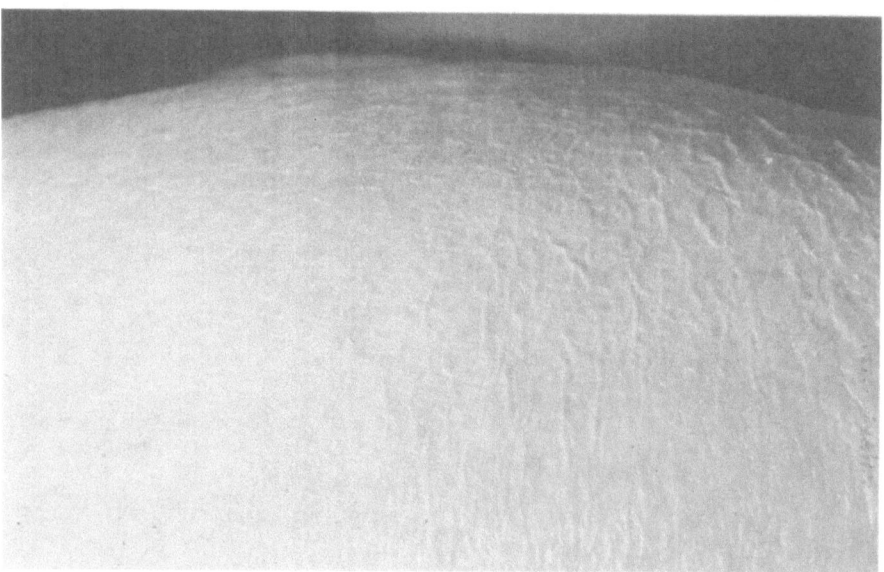

Figure 9.3 Eczema craquelé

The skin as an immunological barrier is dealt with elsewhere (see Chapter 6). I will therefore concentrate on the skin as a barrier to chemical irritants. An irritant is 'any agent capable of producing skin damage if applied for sufficient time and in sufficient concentration'. There is a continuum of intensity of clinical reaction between that of a chemical burn, an irritant dermatitis, and a mild non-eczematous irritant reaction. Dermatitis only occurs when the repair capacity of the skin is exhausted or when penetration of chemicals through the stratum corneum excites an inflammatory response.

The most plausible hypothesis as to how the skin protects itself against irritants is that proposed by Malten[2]. He postulates that each individual has a certain 'metabolic' stratum corneum reserve or repair capacity and that dermatitis only develops when this reserve has been exhausted. The 'repair capacity' may be overrun by one single excessive exposure to an irritant. More commonly, dermatitis is the result of a series of irritants leading to the eventual development of a cumulative, irritant contact dermatitis. Individuals will, of course, vary in their metabolic reserve and therefore their resistance to chemical attack[3]. The speed at which individuals can repair the stratum corneum barrier is also a constant factor and therefore the time taken for recovery following severe irritant dermatitis is always longer than that from a mild or trivial insult.

Even though the mechanisms of allergic and irritant dermatitis are apparently so dissimilar, it is puzzling to know why it is often so difficult to differentiate allergic from irritant reactions, either clinically, histologically or on patch testing. The only sure way remains the testing of chemicals in a dose-response sequence in the affected individual compared with a control population. In an attempt to explore this phenomenon in more detail, we have recently conducted a sequential study comparing contact irritant and contact allergic dermatitis in human volunteers using both conventional microscopy, immunocytochemistry and transmission electronmicroscopy[4] with biopsy times extending from 3 hours to 7 days. We were unable to find any histological or immunocytochemical difference between dermatitis induced by irritants and that due to re-exposure to known allergens. Although the trigger may be different, the immunological/inflammatory response would appear to be the same for both types of attack.

Finally, although we tend to lump all irritants together as though they are an homogenous group, it is obvious that this is far from true. Individual irritants vary in the nature of their attack on the skin, both clinically (seen particularly well by macro-photography) and histologically, which partly explains the variable cellular infiltrates reported in different series in irritant contact dermatitis. They also vary in respect to their damaging effect on the stratum corneum which can now be studied by techniques such as transepidermal water loss measurement. It is likely therefore that the response of the skin to irritants will soon be given the attention that it deserves.

REFERENCES

1. Barry, B.W. (1983). Dermatological Formulations: Percutaneous Absorption. (New York: Marcel Dekker Inc.)
2. Malten, K.E. (1981). Thoughts on irritant contact dermatitis. Contact Dermatitis, **7**, 238
3. Malten, K.E. and den Arend, J.A. (1985). Irritant contact dermatitis. Traumiterative and cumulative impairment by cosmetics, climate, and other daily loads. Derm. Beruf. Umwelt., **33**(4), 125
4. Willis, C.M., Young, E., Brandon, D.R. and Wilkinson, J.D. (1986). Immunopathological and ultrastructural findings in human allergic and irritant contact dermatitis. Br. J. Dermatol., **115**, 305

Section III

INTERFACIAL INTERACTIONS

Chapter 10

A critical review of percutaneous penetration studies

M I Foreman

As is evident from the variety of topics covered in this book, skin, as an organ, performs a number of diverse functions. One is to control the transport of physiologically important material to and from the body, and to prevent so far as possible the ingress of foreign substances. It is this role of skin as a barrier which is of prime interest here. Studies in this area contribute to the further understanding of the structure and function of skin, and have the additional practical importance that transdermal drug delivery has in some circumstances attractive advantages over other methods of drug administration[1].

In this context, the ideal would be the ability to predict, for any given drug molecule, the rate of skin penetration, and the effects of excipient materials, moisture, temperature, humidity, disease, etc. Despite a great deal of research, however, this remains an elusive goal. Even with simple molecules, prospective judgement in all but the broadest sense cannot yet replace practical study of each case. Present knowledge cannot yet accurately predict the penetrative abilities of new molecules. There sometimes even seems to be a Law of Dermatology to the effect that, to any drug with therapeutic potential, for which transdermal delivery offers major advantages, the skin will present an almost impenetrable barrier. The converse is that, where a compound is not required to penetrate skin, it will in fact do so readily, and will, furthermore, produce an unwanted adverse reaction. This represents an admittedly jaundiced view, deliberately slanted to emphasize the point that problems still remain to be overcome. Fortunately too, the first statement of the above 'Law' does not apply in the case of many dermatoses, where the disease itself impairs the skin barrier and facilitates local drug penetration.

Research into the barrier function of skin has been carried out over a range of disciplines, from pharmacology to physical chemistry. In pharmacological terms, the end-organ response following application of a pharmacologically active agent to the skin has provided insight into various aspects of the skin as a barrier membrane. The vasoconstriction induced by corticosteroids applied to skin, which can be seen as a local blanching and assessed at least semiquantitatively, is the prime example[2,3]. Such studies have been of major benefit in designing improved formulations for transdermal corticosteroid delivery[4]. Other examples include the local erythema produced by nicotinic acid and its derivatives[5].

The situation with the corticosteroids, where the drug induces a rapid, easily visualized, local response, was particularly fortuitous. In other instances, studies of drug penetration have needed to employ end-organ responses rather more 'remote' from the skin, or have monitored blood or tissue levels of the drug. Such approaches frequently monitor responses of sites 'remote' spatially, or remote in the sense that drug metabolism intervenes between the application and the measured parameter. More comprehensive pharmacokinetic models, in which transport across the skin is treated as a discrete factor, have been developed in specific cases[6].

Using these various approaches, it can be demonstrated that skin is not impermeable, as once thought, and that the barrier property resides largely in the thin outer skin layer, the stratum corneum[7]. Mechanical damage to this layer greatly accelerates the penetration of material through the skin[8]. Impairment of the barrier can also be achieved by excessive stratum corneum hydration[9].

Whether approached via pharmacology, pharmacokinetics or purely as a problem in physical chemistry, the complexity of skin presents formidable problems. It consists broadly of three layers, the stratum corneum, the viable epidermis and the dermis, each being inhomogeneous, and very different from its neighbour. It is a living organ, constantly changing, and this has consequences for its role as a barrier. It is multifunctional, and it is also the case that structures within skin which subserve various functions may compromise the barrier. This is particularly true of the follicular orifices discussed further below[10-12].

THE USUAL ASSUMPTIONS

Inevitably therefore, both qualitative and quantitative approaches to the measurement of the barrier function have been based on a number of simplifying assumptions. At this stage of development, progress may best be characterized in terms of the number of such assumptions which may be abandoned.

For example, it is inherent in many pharmacological and pharmacokinetic approaches that the skin is treated as a single homogeneous entity. This is patently not so, and there is no single route by which applied material may cross the skin. There has been considerable discussion, for example, of the contribution of hair follicles towards transdermal penetration. The effective surface area of the follicular openings is small in comparison to the total surface area of the skin[13], so that this 'accelerated' route of penetration may be relatively unimportant. Nevertheless, when considering the penetration of various components of crude coal tar into the skin, as shown in Figure 10.1, it is difficult to avoid the conclusion that the follicular apparatus has played a significant role[14].

It is, however, generally accepted that the barrier layer in normal skin resides almost exclusively in the stratum corneum. Mechanical damage to this layer can greatly accelerate the passage of material through the skin. The general assumption, therefore,

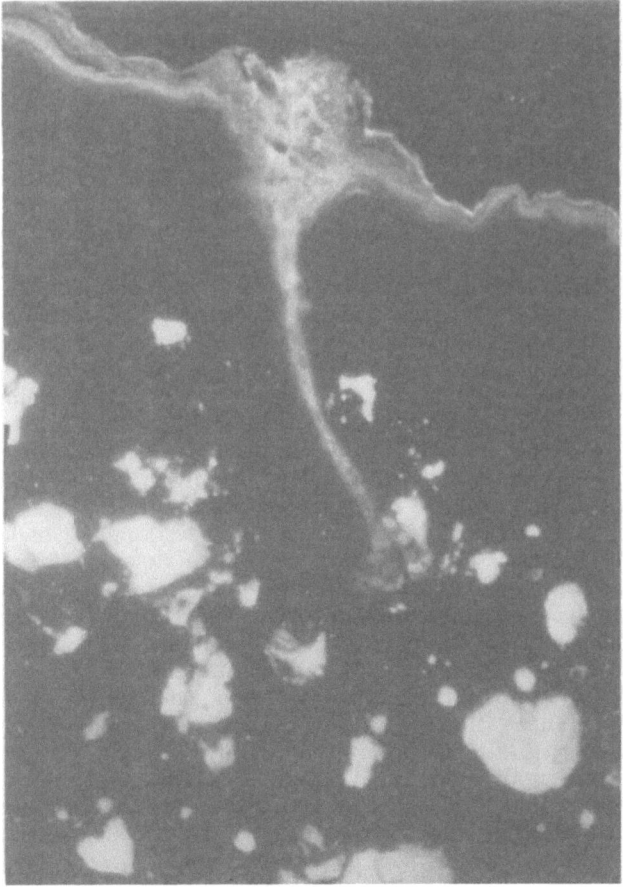

Figure 10.1 Unstained, unfixed section of hairless hamster skin following application of crude coal tar to the skin surface, viewed under ultraviolet light. Components of the tar are evident throughout the follicular duct and in specific areas
within the dermis

that the skin may be regarded as comprising a single layer, so far
as its barrier function is concerned, is in most cases valid. There
may be circumstances where the contribution of the other skin
layers should also be considered[15], but these probably only rarely
occur in practice.

Physicochemical studies of the barrier have the advantage of
studying the passage of diffusing material more directly. They are
most appropriate to in vitro investigations, where the usual
reservation, that an organ in vitro is hardly the same as in vivo,
may not apply, since the prime barrier, the stratum corneum, is
essentially a 'dead' layer. Many substances, hydrocortisone is one
well-known example[16], are extensively metabolized by skin.
However, general metabolic activity mostly resides in the epidermis

and dermal appendages such as the sebaceous gland, and not in the stratum corneum, although the stratum corneum of the sole is an exception[17]. The assumption that the stratum corneum comprises the only penetration barrier removes the immediate need for concern about what happens to the material after it passes this layer, so far as straightforward diffusion studies are concerned.

A much more serious and less valid assumption has been widely adopted in physicochemical studies of skin. It is the main aim of such studies to obtain fundamental, quantitative information concerning the diffusion or migration of material within the stratum corneum. This means, in effect, the determination of diffusion constants, bringing the mathematics of diffusion into the problem[18]. Even in simple systems, diffusion mathematics is complex, with the result that only a limited range of experimental designs yield data from which the diffusion constant for the substance under investigation may be conveniently extracted. The approach most commonly employed is based on a solution of the diffusion problem by Daynes[19]. This solution was first described in 1920, and was applied to the problem of gaseous diffusion across a rubber membrane, being more concerned with how long a balloon could remain inflated than with diffusion processes in skin. This approach has subsequently been used extensively in skin penetration studies. Although it has provided an essential basis for understanding the subject, primarily in the hands of Scheuplein, it suffers from the great disadvantage that the experiment must be carried out with the skin sample mounted between two solutions (usually aqueous). Under these circumstances the skin rapidly becomes saturated with water. A prior assumption of this approach, therefore, is that such a degree of skin hydration as is achieved under these circumstances is unimportant, and the diffusion data so obtained are quoted as if applicable to non-hydrated 'normal' skin. This assumption is greatly at odds with evidence gained over many years which suggests that the barrier property of skin is critically dependent on its level of hydration.

Occlusion of skin, by applying a water impermeable covering, increases the level of stratum corneum hydration, and enhances the penetration of material applied beneath the occlusive film[9]. On this basis many drugs for transdermal delivery are formulated in water resistant excipients and occlusive tapes[20] to facilitate their penetration. The effect can be dramatically demonstrated by corticosteroid-induced vasoconstriction, which is enhanced several fold if the material is applied under occlusion.

THE RESERVOIR

Vickers has demonstrated a further characteristic effect of hydration on the stratum corneum barrier[21]. From experiments, again with corticosteroid-induced vasoconstriction, the presence of a drug 'reservoir' within the stratum corneum can be demonstrated. Transient applications of a corticosteroid to the skin will induce an apparent vasoconstriction which will in due time disappear. Subsequent re-occlusion of the original application site results in a re-appearance of the vasoconstrictor response. Observations of this kind have been interpreted as showing that a proportion of the originally applied corticosteroid has been immobilized within the stratum corneum. Re-occlusion subsequently releases this material which then induces a second vasoconstriction response.

There is a very large body of evidence to show that stratum corneum hydration has a fundamental effect on the skin as a barrier. The removal, in physicochemical studies, of the need to ignore this factor, is therefore a major advance[22,23]. An approach has been described, based on computer simulation of the diffusion process, which allows diffusion in skin in vitro to be studied under circumstances where one surface is open to the atmosphere[24]. In such a case, the level of stratum corneum hydration is likely to be similar to that found under normal in vivo circumstances. The effect of occlusion on the diffusion process may now be directly studied by covering the skin in this arrangement with a water impermeable plastic sheet. There is sufficient flexibility in this approach, not only to study diffusion in skin which is more 'normal', but to study in physicochemical terms the effect of hydration itself. It also opens up possibilities for more easily comprehended methods for comparing the penetrative abilities of different molecules in skin[15].

Using this technique, the presence of the stratum corneum reservoir is immediately apparent. Figure 10.2 shows diffusion curves for the steroid nandrolone calculated from published diffusion parameters for this molecule in occluded and non-occluded skin. It is evident that the diffusion process is tending to a limit appreciably less than the total amount of steroid initially applied to the skin surface. This limit is approached much more closely, however, if the skin is occluded by a plastic film. The most immediate explanation of this effect is that a proportion of the applied steroid has been retained within the stratum corneum 'reservoir' described by Vickers, and that the capacity of the reservoir is greatly diminished by occlusion. The effect is illustrated perhaps more effectively in Figure 10.3, which shows the effect of occluding the skin sample 75 hours after application of the diffusing material. There is a dramatic change in the shape of the diffusion curve as the material previously bound within the stratum corneum reservoir is released.

It would appear therefore that at least two mechanisms are involved in the stratum corneum barrier. Firstly, the process of diffusion within the stratum corneum is slow, and secondly, a proportion of the diffusing material is effectively immobilized within this layer. Both mechanisms appear to be affected by hydration. From Table 10.1 it may be seen that the diffusion rate, as measured by the diffusion constant, is increased in hydrated skin. And, as already indicated, the fraction of diffusing material retained within the stratum corneum is diminished.

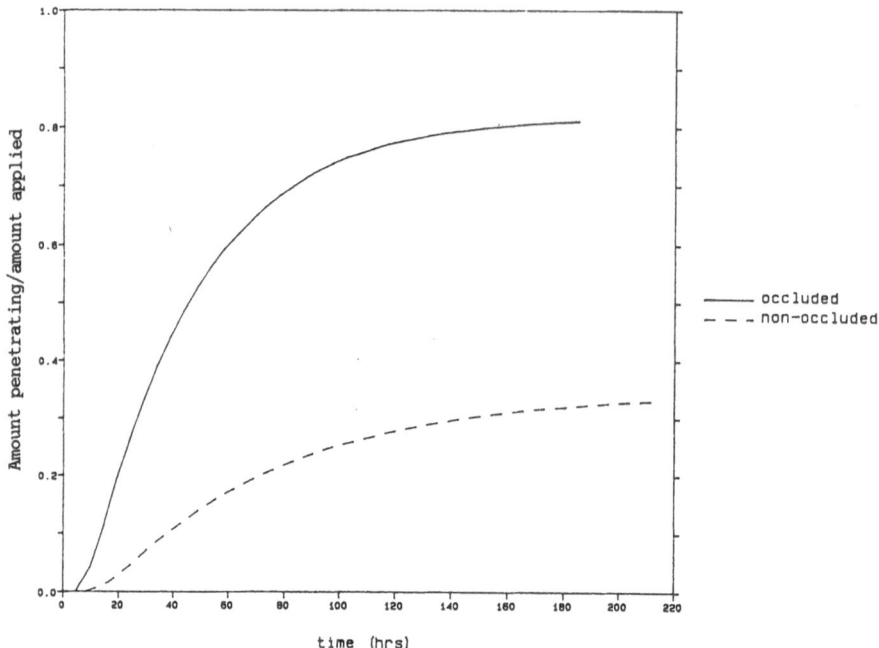

Figure 10.2 Diffusion curves for nandrolone in occluded and non-occluded human skin, calculated from the diffusion constants and bound fractions of reference 26

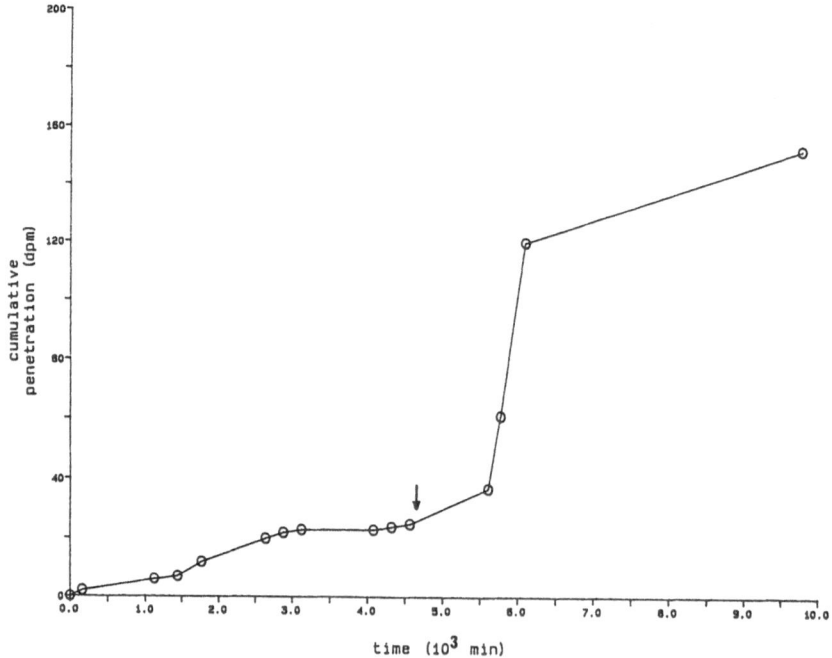

Figure 10.3 Diffusion of nandrolone in a single piece of human skin, initially open to the air at 22 ± 2°C, plastic film occlusion being applied after 75 hours (arrow)

86

Table 10.1 Diffusion parameters for various steroids in whole human skin at 22 ± 2°C

Steroid		Diffusion constant D $(m^2 s^{-1})$	Bound fraction F
Nandrolone	non-occluded	$3.2 \pm 0.5 \times 10^{-12}$	0.35 ± 0.05
	occluded	$4.9 \pm 0.7 \times 10^{-12}$	0.82 ± 0.06
Rimexolone	non-occluded	$7.9 \pm 0.6 \times 10^{-13}$	0.34 ± 0.08
	occluded	$2.6 \pm 0.9 \times 10^{-12}$	0.75 ± 0.15
Corticosterone	non-occluded	$9.9 \pm 1.4 \times 10^{-13}$	0.42 ± 0.06
	occluded	$1.4 \pm 0.3 \times 10^{-13}$	0.85 ± 0.06
Triamcinolone acetonide	non-occluded	$7.6 \pm 1.1 \times 10^{-13}$	0.39 ± 0.04
	occluded	$1.4 \pm 0.3 \times 10^{-12}$	0.83 ± 0.06

Data of reference 26. Values are means ± SEM
Rimexolone (Organon): 11β-hydroxy-16α,17α,21-trimethylpregna-1,4-diene-3,20-dione

More fundamental understanding would be forthcoming from a knowledge of the energies involved in the diffusion and reservoir-binding processes. Again, the complexity of skin presents considerable problems in obtaining such information. In general, measurement of the energies involved in any physical process requires a study of the system over as wide a range of temperature as possible. Changes occur within the stratum corneum, however, as the temperature changes[25]. Most obviously, phase changes occur in epidermal lipid, which limit the temperature ranges over which meaningful measurement can be made. Further restrictions may be imposed by other temperature-dependent processes. However, one attempt has been made to assess the temperature dependence and thereby the energies involved in the diffusion and reservoir-binding phenomena[26]. For the diffusion of nandrolone in stratum corneum, the activation energy for the diffusion process was found to be 26 ± 9 kJ/mol. This is not a particularly high value, and may indicate that this molecule traverses the stratum corneum by moving between rather than through squames which make up the majority of the stratum corneum (route A rather than B in Figure 10.4). For the latter route the activation energy might be expected to be much higher. The slowness of the diffusion process in this instance may well be a consequence of the tortuosity of the route traversed.

The stratum corneum reservoir, on the other hand, may be envisaged as a set of binding sites within the stratum corneum, to which water is normally bound. Certain molecules diffusing within the skin may disperse water from these sites, and become bound themselves. This process may be reversed only if water is present in large excess, when the skin is occluded for example. Approached in this way, it has been shown that the fraction of bound material changes in a manner consistent with the above model, and that the energy required for displacement of water from the bound sites is 60 ± 11 kJ/mol. This energy requirement is less than would be

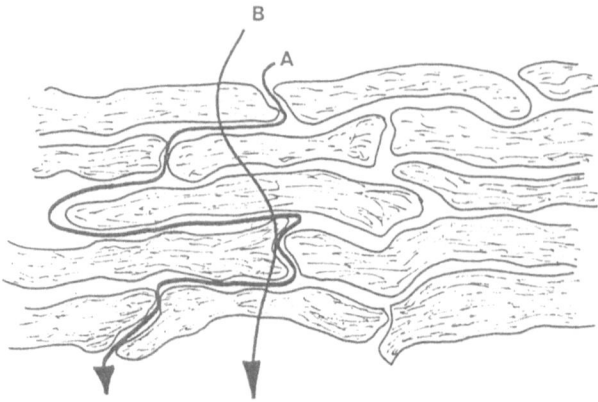

Figure 10.4 Major routes of diffusion within the stratum corneum. A: Intercorneocyte route; B: Transcorneocyte route

encountered in a case of covalent chemical bonding, but more than for a simple adsorption process[26]. It is more similar to chemisorption processes, such as the adsorption of unsaturated polyene hydrocarbons onto activated charcoal.

It seems probable that binding within the stratum corneum reservoir has an essential role to play in the function of skin as a barrier. In vitro the reservoir may be studied as an essentially static process, and the energies involved may be measured. In the living animal however, the process is dynamic. Material immobilized within the reservoir will be discarded as the stratum corneum is sloughed off as part of the ongoing process of epidermal turnover, part of the 'external loss' of the applied material[27]. Such an active role of living skin in the prevention of ingress of foreign material is intuitively very appealing, and investigations which combine studies of diffusion within skin with epidermal turnover and the rate at which the stratum corneum is discarded may represent the next major advance in this field.

REFERENCES

1. Barry, B.W. (1983). Dermatological Formulations, Percutaneous Absorption. (New York, Basel: Dekker)
2. McKenzie, A.W. and Stoughton, R.B. (1962). Method for comparing percutaneous absorption of steroids. Arch. Dermatol., **86**, 608-10
3. Clanachan, I., Devitt, H.G., Foreman, M.I. and Kelly, I.P. (1980). The human vasoconstrictor assay for topical steroids. J. Pharmacol. Methods, **4**, 209-20
4. Barry, B.W. and Woodford, R. (1986). The vasoconstrictor test as a model for developing topical formulations. In (eds.) Marks, R. and Plewig, G. Skin Models. pp 103-12. (Berlin: Springer Verlag)
5. Stoughton, R.B., Clendenning, W.E. and Kruse, D. (1960). Percutaneous absorption of nicotinic acid and derivatives. J. Invest. Dermatol., **35**, 337-41
6. Guy, R.H., Hadgraft, J. and Maibach, H.I. (1982). A pharmacokinetic model for percutaneous absorption. Int. J. Pharm., **11**, 119-24
7. Scheuplein, R.J. and Blank, I.H. (1973). Mechanisms of percutaneous absorption. IV. Penetration of non-electrolytes (alcohols) from aqueous solutions and from pure liquids. J. Invest. Dermatol., **66**, 286-96

8. Washitake, M., Yajima, T., Anmo, T., Arita, T. and Hori, R. (1973). Studies on percutaneous absorption of drugs. III. Percutaneous absorption of drugs through damaged skin. Chem. Pharm. Bull., 21, 2444-51

9. Takeda, Y. (1975). An autoradiographic study on the percutaneous absorption of a topical corticosteroid with reference to the effects of occlusion and stripping. J. Dermatol., 2, 131-6

10. Tregear, R.T. (1961). Relative penetrability of hair follicles and epidermis. J. Physiol., 156, 307-13

11. Scheuplein, R.J. (1967). Mechanism of percutaneous absorption. II. Transient diffusion and the relative importance of various routes of skin penetration. J. Invest. Dermatol., 48, 79-88

12. Scheuplein, R.J. (1972). Properties of the skin as a membrane. In (eds.) Stoughton, R.B. and Van Scott, E.J. Pharmacology and the Skin. Chap. X, pp 125-52. (New York: Appleton-Century-Crofts)

13. Scheuplein, R.J. and Blank, I.H. (1971). Permeability of the skin. Physiol. Rev., 51, 702-47

14. Foreman, M.I., Picton, W., Lukowiecki, G.A. and Clark, C. (1979). The effect of topical crude coal tar on unstimulated hairless hamster skin. Br. J. Dermatol., 100, 707-15

15. Foreman, M.I., Clanachan, I. and Kelly, I.P. (1983). Diffusion barriers in skin, a new method of comparison. Br. J. Dermatol., 108, 549-53

16. Hsia, S.L. and Lee, H.Y. (1966). Metabolic transformations of cortisol-4-^{14}C in human skin. Biochemistry, 5, 1469-74

17. Hershey, F.B., Lewis Jr., C., Murphy, J. and Schiff, T. (1960). Quantitative histochemistry of human skin. J. Histochem. Cytochem., 8, 41-9

18. Crank, J. (1970). The Mathematics of Diffusion. (Oxford: Oxford University Press)

19. Daynes, H. (1920). The process of diffusion through a rubber membrane. Proc. R. Soc., A97, 286-307

20. Berger, J.E. and Helm, F. (1970). Flurandrenolone tape. New means of achieving occlusive therapy. N. Y. State J. Med., 70, 406-8

21. Vickers, C.F.H. (1963). Existence of a reservoir in the stratum corneum - experimental proof. Arch. Dermatol., 88, 20-5

22. Scheuplein, R.J. and Ross, L.W. (1974). Mechanism of percutaneous absorption. V. Percutaneous absorption of solvent deposited solids. J. Invest. Dermatol., 62, 353-60

23. Foreman, M.I. (1986). Stratum corneum hydration; consequences for skin permeation experiments. Drug. Dev. Ind. Pharm., 12, 461-3

24. Foreman, M.I., Kelly, I. and Lukowiecki, G.A. (1977). A method for the measurement of diffusion constants suitable for studies of non-occluded skin. J. Pharm. Pharmacol., 29, 108-9

25. Van Duzee, B.F. (1975). Thermal analysis of human stratum corneum. J. Invest. Dermatol., 65, 404-8

26. Foreman, M.I. and Clanachan, I. (1984). Steroid diffusion and binding in human stratum corneum. J. Chem. Soc. Faraday Trans., 1, 80, 3439-44

27. Feldman, R.J. and Maibach, H.I. (1965). Penetration of ^{14}C-hydrocortisone through normal skin. Arch. Dermatol., 91, 661-6

Chapter 11

Percutaneous absorption: transdermal drug delivery systems

B W Barry

PHILOSOPHY OF TRANSDERMAL ADMINISTRATION

Transdermal drug delivery systems are topical devices designed originally to deliver a potent drug to the surface of the skin at a controlled rate. This rate was intended to be well below the maximum that human skin can accept. Thus, the fundamental concept of this novel dosage form was that the device, and not the stratum corneum, should control the flux of drug diffusing through the epidermis and dermis and passing into the general circulation via the capillaries.

The original Transdermal Therapeutic System (TTS, Transderm or Transiderm) of the Alza Corporation aimed to provide prophylactic systemic therapy for acute or chronic conditions in a more effective, convenient way than parenteral or oral therapy. Thus, skin administration eliminates variables which influence gastrointestinal absorption, such as pH changes, food intake, stomach emptying time and intestinal motility and transit time. The topical route bypasses the liver, avoiding first-pass metabolism, although we should remember that viable skin tissues also contain enzymes capable of efficiently attacking drug molecules as they pass in high dilution across the skin. Transdermal input may provide controlled, constant drug administration and thus allow only one pharmacological effect to dominate from a drug which, in a conventional dosage form, shows several effects. For drugs with short half-lives this continuity of input may ensure constant plasma concentrations which are difficult to obtain orally; enhanced patient compliance is an added advantage. Peaks in plasma drug concentrations often cause unpleasant side-effects but controlled entry eliminates pulsing in the systemic circulation. This control is also valuable for drugs with a narrow therapeutic index. Although it is claimed that if the patient needs to terminate therapy rapidly, simple removal of the device will interrupt absorption we should remember that the stratum corneum can serve as a reservoir for many agents and thus provide a prolonged, but steadily decreasing, trickle of medicament to the viable tissues[1].

DEVICE DESIGN AND IN VITRO PERFORMANCES

This chapter deals only with selected aspects of the design and preclinical in vitro testing of transdermal devices; the approach used owes much to the excellent article by Good[2].

If we accept for the moment the basic, initial philosophy on which transdermal systems were introduced to medicine (that the skin acts as a perfect sink for the permeating drug molecules), we can identify two main designs for these devices, the monolithic or matrix system and the patch which incorporates a rate-limiting membrane.

In the monolithic system no rate-controlling membrane separates the drug reservoir from the sink and the drug concentration in the device decreases with time. The general shape of the cumulative release curve follows the Higuchi 'square root of time' law (Figure 11.1). For a membrane-controlled device, such as the Alza Transderm, Figure 11.2 illustrates the delivery profile when the rate-controlling membrane is initially free of the drug. The intercept

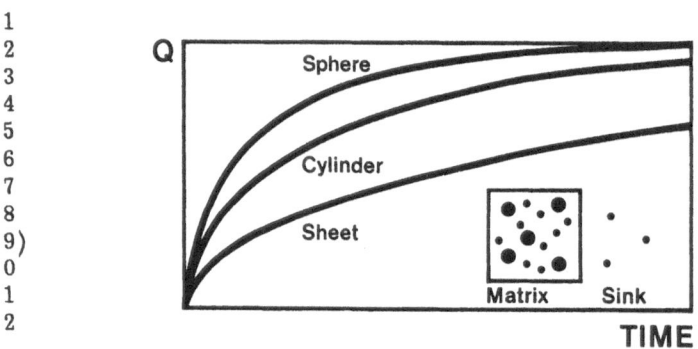

Figure 11.1 Cumulative amount released (Q) versus time for various geometries with 'sheet' representing matrix device used transdermally. Inset shows a device releasing into a sink with large circles (drug particles) providing dissolved, diffusing drug molecules (small dots)

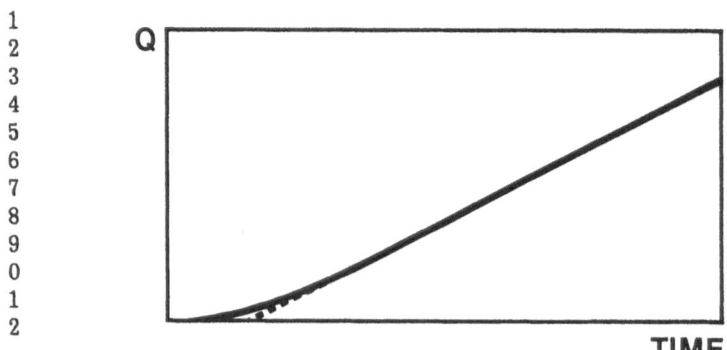

Figure 11.2 Cumulative release profile for a membrane controlled system with membrane initially free of drug

indicates that time is required for the drug concentration in the membrane to come to equilibrium with respect to that in the reservoir. However, during storage of a membrane device, the membrane (and the adhesive) will attain an equilibrium concentration of the drug with respect to that in the reservoir (Figure 11.3). At such time, the chemical potentials of the drug in the various layers of the device become equal. The drug in the membrane and adhesive is more readily available to the sink and it produces a 'burst' effect. This burst is greater the higher the concentration of drug in the membrane and adhesive (Figure 11.4).

DELIVERY DEVICE -'PATCH'

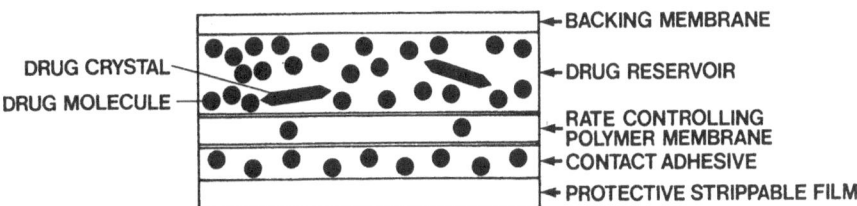

Figure 11.3   Representation of a membrane device showing situation at storage equilibrium

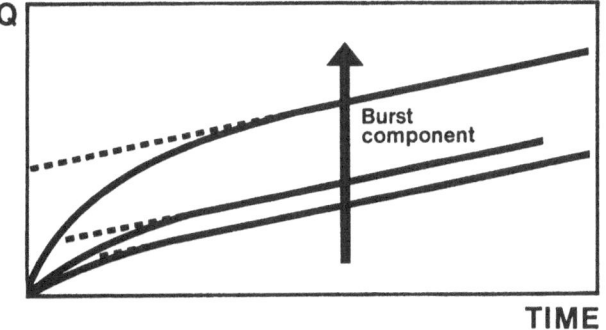

Figure 11.4 Cumulative release profile for membrane-controlled systems with burst effect - modified from Good[2]

Transdermal scopolamine (hyoscine)

The first membrane device used clinically consisted of a thin, multilayered disc for placing behind the ear, a relatively permeable skin site in humans. The system delivers hyoscine (scopolamine) for the treatment of motion sickness. In the usual dosage form of injections or tablets, hyoscine can induce confusion, excitement and even hallucinations; the controlled low-level input of the drug from the Transderm aims to eliminate these effects. Two-thirds of its users still experience a dry mouth, but even this has been turned to advantage by a recorder-playing physician who found that a patch rapidly suppressed salivation.

The hyoscine patch went into space with American astronauts, it can control radiation sickness and the side-effects of anti-cancer drug treatment, but its main users are the travelling public. Prominent display of the device even provides a status symbol for holiday makers about to leave on their world cruises!

Transdermal nitroglycerin

A second major use of patch technology is to deliver nitroglycerin and other nitrates for the treatment of angina, congestive heart failure and acute myocardial infarction. At present (1985) there is much dispute about the relative merits of the various nitroglycerin transdermal devices, ointments and tablets. The main arguments revolve around whether or not the patch systems deliver suboptimal drug levels, whether tolerance develops to the drug, or if the device rather than the patient's skin (with its inherent inter- and intrasubject variability in permeability) controls the drug input. The question regarding suboptimal drug levels will probably have to be answered by clinical usage, although one comment often offered by patients is that the patch stimulates low-grade, constant headaches in place of the periodic, splitting headache of buccal treatment. It appears that in the USA, in defiance of the suspicions of physicians, many patients are keen patch users, the phenomenon being referred to as discomania[3]. An answer as to whether or not tolerance develops after 24-hour use (as claimed by some investigations) is complicated by the fact that in most (or all?) long-term clinical trials, patients may also take glyceryl trinitrate tablets when they deem it necessary. The patient will then experience 'spiking' of the plasma concentration.

The question as to exactly where is the rate-limiting step in the overall process of percutaneous absorption from a patch is a fundamental one, of clinical relevance and not only of scientific interest. Our assumption up until now has been that the skin functions as a perfect sink, but how true is this for nitroglycerin? The skin is a particularly complex organ, but within this multilayered tissue it is clear that for most drugs, including nitroglycerin, the stratum corneum represents the prime barrier to drug transport. As is also common, there are large intersubject variabilities in glyceryl trinitrate transport with a mean value quoted of approximately 25 μg cm^{-2} h^{-1} using cadaver skin at 32°C. Values of less than 7 and greater than 50 μg cm^{-2} h^{-1} are not uncommon.

At present, there are several transdermal nitroglycerin patches on the market (Table 11.1).

The Transderm-Nitro has the typical structure of a membrane-controlled device developed using the Alza technology. Within a few hours after manufacture, nitroglycerin equilibrates according to its relative solubility into both the adhesive and the control membrane.

94

Table 11.1 Transdermal nitroglycerin devices

Name	Company	Type
Transderm-Nitro	Ciba-Geigy	membrane
Nitrodisc	Searle	matrix
Nitro-Dur	Key	matrix
Deponit	Pharma-Schwarz	matrix/multilayer

Thus, we would expect that the release of nitroglycerin in vitro should resemble that from a membrane system with an initial burst effect. Figure 11.5 illustrates the release profile for Transderm-Nitro into an infinite sink of water. Three regions with different boundary conditions are evident - the burst effect at short times, the steady state flux through the rate-controlling membrane and the depletion region operating at long times when sufficient nitroglycerin has left the device to reduce its system concentration below saturation.

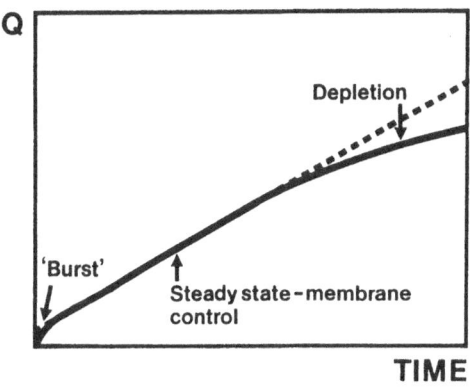

Figure 11.5 Cumulative release profile of nitroglycerin from Transderm-Nitro into infinite sink - modified from Good[2]

However, applying the Transderm-Nitro device to human skin presents an intervening rate process between diffusion of the drug in the device and partitioning into the skin, and elimination from the body. Unfortunately for the theorist, the manufacturer, the physician and not least the patient, the stratum corneum **does** offer a finite resistance to drug permeation and the skin does not act as a perfect sink. A useful theoretical approach is to view the skin/device combinations as a double membrane composed of the system membrane and the horny layer, ignoring the negligible barrier resistance provided by the adhesive.

The next step is to select a range of skin fluxes between 7 and 15 μg cm^{-2} h^{-1} and to compare the predicted absorption profiles from Transderm-Nitro through skin types ranging in permeability from 7 to 150 μg cm^{-2} h^{-1} (Figure 11.6). It is clear that the duration of constant absorption rate depends upon skin permeability. This conclusion is even more relevant for monolithic devices which have no in-built rate-control mechanism. Thus, we can conclude that the Transderm-Nitro only exerts some influence on the net flux or absorption of the drug. The influence of the system's membrane is most readily apparent for highly permeable skin, when the rate-controlling factor is allied more to the device membrane than to stratum corneum permeability. The Transderm-Nitro provides an upper limit to absorption rates for nitroglycerin as revealed by the flux under sink conditions.

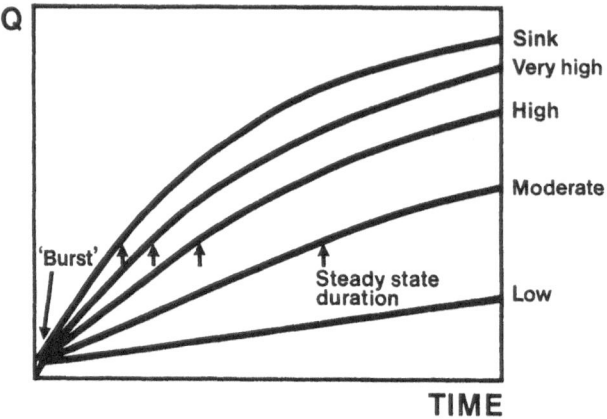

Figure 11.6 Theoretical cumulative absorption profiles for nitroglycerin from Transderm-Nitro through human skin with indicated permeabilities to nitroglycerin - modified from Good[2]

If we turn to a pharmacokinetic treatment for further clarification of the effects of system design, we can note that the appropriate analysis of transdermally applied drugs is, in principle, simple. We can use the one compartment system under constant rate infusion to model the absorption and elimination of nitroglycerin via the plasma. The analysis can cope with the burst effect, steady state delivery and decreasing rate regimen. One analysis for Transderm-Nitro expresses the relevant equations in terms of the temporal fluctuations in the amount of drug in the central compartment and ignores distribution volume terms. Thus, the purpose is qualitatively to illustrate theoretical plasma profiles for different skin permeabilities. The analysis uses a half-life for nitroglycerin of 5 min; Figure 11.7 illustrates the effect of skin permeability on predicted plasma profiles for an applied Transderm-Nitro patch.

These profiles reveal two significant features - the effect which skin permeability has on the magnitude of plasma concentrations and

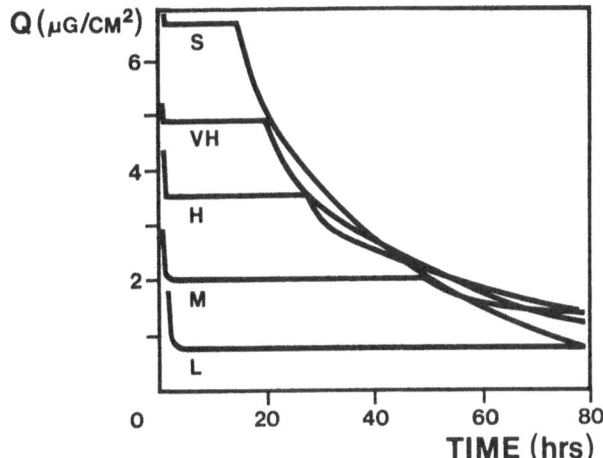

Figure 11.7 Theoretical plasma profiles for nitroglycerin delivered from Transderm-Nitro through skin of permeabilities as represented in Figure 11.6 - modified from Good[2]

the duration of steady-state plasma levels. These effects are even more dramatically illustrated if we compare projected profiles arising from a membrane device with those generated by a monolithic system having only skin control of absorption. We can compare the theoretical plasma profiles generated across skin of low permeability with those from tissue with high permeability (Figure 11.8). For the former, steady-state levels and duration are nearly identical for both systems, but highly permeable skin clearly limits the duration of steady state and generates quite high plasma levels for a device lacking any membrane control.

The argument presented by Ciba-Geigy is that for patients with a highly permeable skin, some system rate control is highly desirable to extend the duration of control and to avoid excessive blood levels. In one of their trials, Ciba-Geigy concluded that rate control was approximately 20-25% system related and 75-80% skin mediated with a fairly high degree of variability.

Practical in vitro experiments which actually compare permeation profiles of nitroglycerin through skin (as distinct from theoretical treatments) tend to use hairless mouse skin. If we accept that hairless mouse skin is an adequate model for human skin - and there are dangers in this approach - the results obtained suggest that even though nitroglycerin may be released into a sink according to different rate profiles from various devices, the drug penetrates through skin according to the same rate process[4].

An idea of the kind of variability met with in practice was provided by a study which investigated the plasma levels obtained in vivo for 12 volunteers comparing TTS-nitroglycerin with a

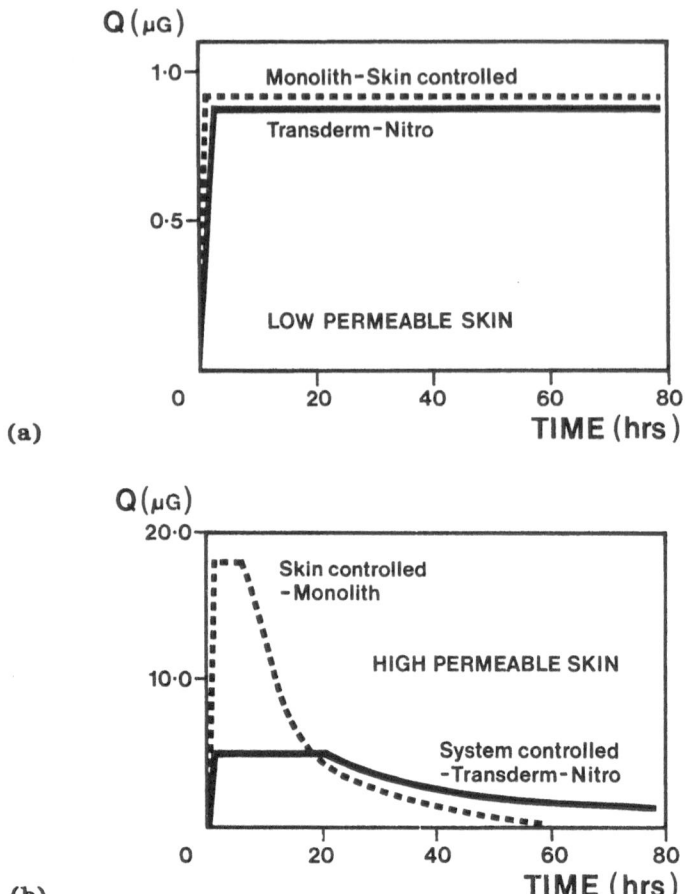

Figure 11.8 Theoretical plasma profiles of nitroglycerin resulting from absorption from a monolithic system (skin controlled) and Transderm-Nitro; **(a)** skin with low permeability **(b)** skin with high permeability - modified from Good[2]

nitroglycerin ointment applied every 8 hours[2]. The ointment seemed quite good!

Nitroglycerin patches have produced some bizarre accidents. This type of patch should be removed before shock electrodes are used to restart the heart after a heart attack - there have been at least four reports of 'explosions' (blue sparking) since Transderm-Nitro was introduced. A doctor recounted his investigation of a man complaining of chest pain and severe headache. The patient's ECG was normal but the physician discovered a patch sticking to the man's abdomen. It seems that the patient's wife used transdermal treatment for her angina and that during the night her patch had dropped off and become attached to her husband, thus accounting for his symptoms. A final example relates to the importance of patient education in respect of the use of novel drug delivery systems. An elderly angina sufferer, enthusiastic over this new mode of treatment, returned to his doctor for help because there was no suitable space available on his skin to which he could attach further patches - no-one had told him to remove the old ones!

THE FUTURE FOR TRANSDERMAL DELIVERY

At various stages of development there are transdermal devices which will deliver, for example, isosorbide dinitrate (for angina), oestradiol for oestrogen replacement therapy in menopausal women, timolol for once-daily β-blocker activity and clonidine for hypertension[5]. The clonidine system (Catapres-TTS) has run into some difficulties. The patch produces sensitivity reactions which the manufacturer thought arose from a sensitizing component in the patch adhesive and which could be removed. However, recent work has revealed a high incidence of local allergic skin reactions to clonidine itself.

Transdermal therapy appears to be on the brink of a rapid expansion for the rate-controlled administration of potent, non-allergenic agents - with suitable physicochemical properties - whose current methods of administration cause problems. However, estimates that by the mid-1990s, 70% or more of all drugs will be delivered by the transdermal patch system owe more to an advertising executive's dreams than to cold reality. Owing to constraints arising from drug potency, stability and physicochemical properties, limited skin permeability and allergic and irritant reactions, I do not believe that transdermal administration will become the preferred dosage form for a high percentage of drugs. There are problems with, for example, cutaneous metabolism and the fact that a relatively small volume of skin has to suffer the entire body load of the drug. The zone between the patch and the skin provides a medium for bacterial and fungal growth with possible subsequent infection as well as microbial metabolism of the drug (surface skin microbial decomposition has already been shown for nitroglycerin). These factors may limit the duration of application of such devices. We know little about the physiological sequelae of long-term occlusions, although the fact that 24-hour patch application may inhibit underlying sweat glands for 72 hours afterwards should provide a note of caution (Maibach, personal communication). There may be problems in the future associated with tissue trauma when patches are removed from the skin.

A fundamental problem with all treatments via percutaneous absorption is the high barrier resistance to permeation of the stratum corneum. One possibility for the future would be to diminish radically this resistance by incorporating into the patch an efficient penetration enhancer such as Azone. We can expect to see a growing interest in the concept of combining potent drugs with active penetration enhancers in transdermal delivery systems.

REFERENCES

1. Barry, B.W. (1983). Dermatological Formulations: Percutaneous Absorption. (New York and Basel: Dekker)
2. Good, W.R. (1983). Transderm-Nitro: controlled delivery of nitroglycerin via the transdermal route. Drug Dev. Ind. Pharm., **9**, 647-70
3. Abrams, J. (1984). The brief saga of transdermal nitroglycerin discs: paradise lost? Am. J. Cardiol., **54**, 220-4
4. Chien, Y.W., Keshary, P.R., Huang, Y.C. and Sarpotdar, P.P. (1983). Comparative controlled skin permeation of nitroglycerin from marketed transdermal delivery systems. J. Pharm. Sci., **72**, 968-70
5. Shaw, J.E. and Mitchell, C. (1983-84). Dermal drug delivery systems: a review. J. Toxicol-Cut. Ocular Toxicol., **2**(4 and 5), 249-66

Chapter 12

Interaction of stratum corneum with water vapour

B B Michniak-Mikolajczak and B W Barry

The stratum corneum or 'cornified layer' is a multicellular, metabolically inactive surface layer of the skin comprised of flattened, stacked cells which are the intact remains of what was once living epidermis tissue. The stratum corneum exhibits regional differences in thickness over the body, being as thick as several hundred micrometres on the palms of the hand and the soles of the feet in adults, the average thickness over the body being about 10 μm. This tissue is also very dense, about 1.5 g cm^{-3} in the dry state[1].

Its cellular origin is in the basal layer of the epidermis where cell division begins a complex process in which cells migrate outward and towards the body surface. In this process the cells flatten and dehydrate and undergo intracellular changes such that, when they become the stratum corneum, they are dense, keratin-filled and metabolically inactive disc-like concentrates of their original forms. In spite of being such a thin membrane, the stratum corneum forms the main barrier to microbes, radiation and chemicals brought into contact with the skin. It is also important as a thermal barrier and as part of the temperature-regulating mechanism.

The general rationale for the use of topical dosage forms involves the manipulation of or assistance of this barrier function of the stratum corneum. The required degree of elasticity of this tissue is dependent upon the proper formation of the stratum corneum (psoriatic plaques tend to split and crack) and on the presence of adequate natural lipids, hygroscopic substances and moisture[2]. Both lipids and water plasticize this tissue, that is, they tend by their presence to make it less brittle and excessive removal of either lipid or moisture leads to 'chapping'. The importance of water in the stratum corneum was first reported by Blank[3] in 1952. He observed that applied oils did not soften the dehydrated stratum corneum, but that water was readily absorbed by the tissue and softened it.

Most determinations on dry skin have been performed using abnormal tissue, such as callus[3], or diseased skin, such as that present in ichthyosis, psoriasis and essential fatty acid deficiency[4-6].

These experiments suggest that such dry skin is thickened, hyperproliferative, depleted in 'natural moisturizing factors', deficient in water-binding capacity, has an abnormal lipid composition and an abnormal permeability to water[7].

Under normal conditions the stratum corneum is always partially hydrated. A gradient in water concentration exists through the tissue corresponding to an average water contentration of approximately 0.90 g g^{-1} dry tissue. This amount of water increases the water permeability of the stratum corneum approximately 10-fold over its value when perfectly dry. Upon additional contact with liquid water the stratum corneum may sorb 3-5 times its own weight[8]. This further hydration results in an additional 2-3-fold increase in the permeability to water and other polar molecules. For example, the flux of cortisone through dry stratum corneum (using a diaphragm cell technique) is about 2.64 x 10^{-11} mol cm^{-2} h^{-1}. After 20 days the drying agent (Drierite) was removed and the stratum corneum was allowed to hydrate and the flux increased to 3.62 x 10^{-11} mol cm^2 h^{-1}. Finally, replacement of the Drierite[9] caused a fall to 2.70 x 10^{-11} mol cm^{-2} h^{-1}. The state of hydration of the stratum corneum has been accepted for some time as of major importance in influencing percutaneous absorption. Wurster and Kramer[10] measured the rate of penetration of esters of salicylic acid through skin with dry and hydrated stratum corneum. They found that when the tissue was hydrated the rate of penetration of the most water-soluble ester increased more than that of the other esters studied. Working with aspirin in a temperature-humidity chamber, Fritsch and Stoughton[11] showed the dual importance of these factors on the penetration of excised skin. Full hydration of the stratum corneum, accomplished by layering water over salicylic acid on the epidermal surface, dramatically increased the penetration compared to conditions of lower humidity at the same temperature. Many methods are available for assessing the level of skin water content and some examples are presented.

IN VIVO METHODS FOR MEASURING SKIN HYDRATION

(1) Transpirometry
     electrohydrometric estimation of water loss
     thermal conductivity
     gravimetry
     infra-red absorption,
(2) Low magnification photography of stratum corneum surface,
(3) Scanning electron microscopy,
(4) Nuclear magnetic resonance.

IN VITRO METHODS OF MEASURING SKIN HYDRATION

(1) Gravimetric measurement,
(2) Differential scanning calorimetry,
(3) Biomechanical analysis - measuring reversible stretching properties,
(4) Diffusion cell techniques using radiolabelled compounds,
(5) Nuclear magnetic resonance.

FACTORS WHICH SHOULD BE CONSIDERED IN EXPERIMENTAL DESIGN

(1) Species - human or animal models,
(2) In vivo or in vitro experiment,
(3) Age,
(4) Regional skin sample site,
(5) Preparation of skin sample and its storage (in vitro),
(6) Skin condition - previous treatment, stripping,
(7) Temperature,
(8) Humidity,
(9) Blood flow (in vivo).

The value of a diffusion coefficient gives information about how fast a substance such as water diffuses through a stratum corneum sample with time. The law governing diffusion is termed Fick's first law of diffusion[12]:

$$J = -D\frac{dc}{dx}$$

where D is the diffusion coefficient for a substance in a medium at a particular temperature and pressure with units of length^2 time^{-1}, dc/dx is the change in concentration c of the diffusing substance across a distance x and J is the amount of substance per unit area flowing per unit time. The negative sign occurs since the diffusion is taking place in the opposite direction to the concentration gradient.

An alternative formulation is:

$$\frac{dc}{dt} = D\frac{d^2c}{dx^2}$$

This is termed Fick's second law of diffusion showing that the rate of diffusion is dependent on the rate of change of the penetrant concentration gradient across a barrier.

Examples of some approximate diffusion coefficients for human stratum corneum[13] are, for liquid water 10^{-9}, progesterone 10^{-11}, cortisone 10^{-12} and hydrocortisone 10^{-13} cm^2 s^{-1}.

Many techniques have been developed to generate information on the type and quantity of water within the stratum corneum, its mobility, and the influence exerted by compounds applied to the corneum on its diffusion characteristics. Two main in vitro techniques were used, the gravimetric method and the diffusion cell method. The former technique has been widely used[8]; however, in this present study it has been improved and extended.

GRAVIMETRIC METHOD OF MEASURING WATER VAPOUR UPTAKE IN STRATUM CORNEUM

Strips of dried human abdominal stratum corneum were suspended in a microbalance chamber, the weight of these samples being displayed on a Robal microprocessor unit to three decimal places in milligrams (Figure 12.1). Dry air was passed through either a drying agent (Drierite) or water and then mixed well (in differing proportions) to produce required relative humidities (RH). For the purposes of these experiments values of 0 and 91% RH were chosen. The humidity was monitored via two humidity sensors and was displayed on a humidity meter. The flow and pressure of the incoming air were controlled and the entire apparatus (in Figure 12.1) was enclosed in a controlled temperature cabinet at 32 ± 0.2°C in a constant-temperature room (22 ± 1°C). Alternatively 0% RH could be produced by suspending the stratum corneum above a glass chamber (Figure 12.2) containing Drierite or 91% with the samples over a saturated solution of potassium nitrate[14]. In these experiments the air flow from the main apparatus was cut off entirely. Water vapour sorption (0-91% RH) and desorption (91-0% RH) patterns were studied recording the weight change in the stratum corneum samples every minute for 24 hours. All data were stored on a computer printout and initial diffusion coefficients were calculated (D_i). The experiments in which air flow was used were termed the flow system and when Drierite or saturated potassium chloride was used to produce the required RH, the stationary system.

Preparation of the stratum corneum samples[15]

(1) Frozen (-20°C) human abdominal skin samples obtained post-mortem were thawed.

(2) Excess fat was scraped off using a razor blade.

(3) Skin was put in water at 60°C for 45 seconds.

(4) Stratum corneum was then peeled off.

(5) Tissue was treated with 0.0001% w/v trypsin and 0.5% w/v sodium bicarbonate for 12 hours at 37°C. This step was omitted for samples used in the diffusion cell technique. Excess epidermis was removed using forceps.

(6) Tissue was spread out on a wire mesh sprayed with PTFE.

(7) The tissue was placed in a desiccator ready for use.

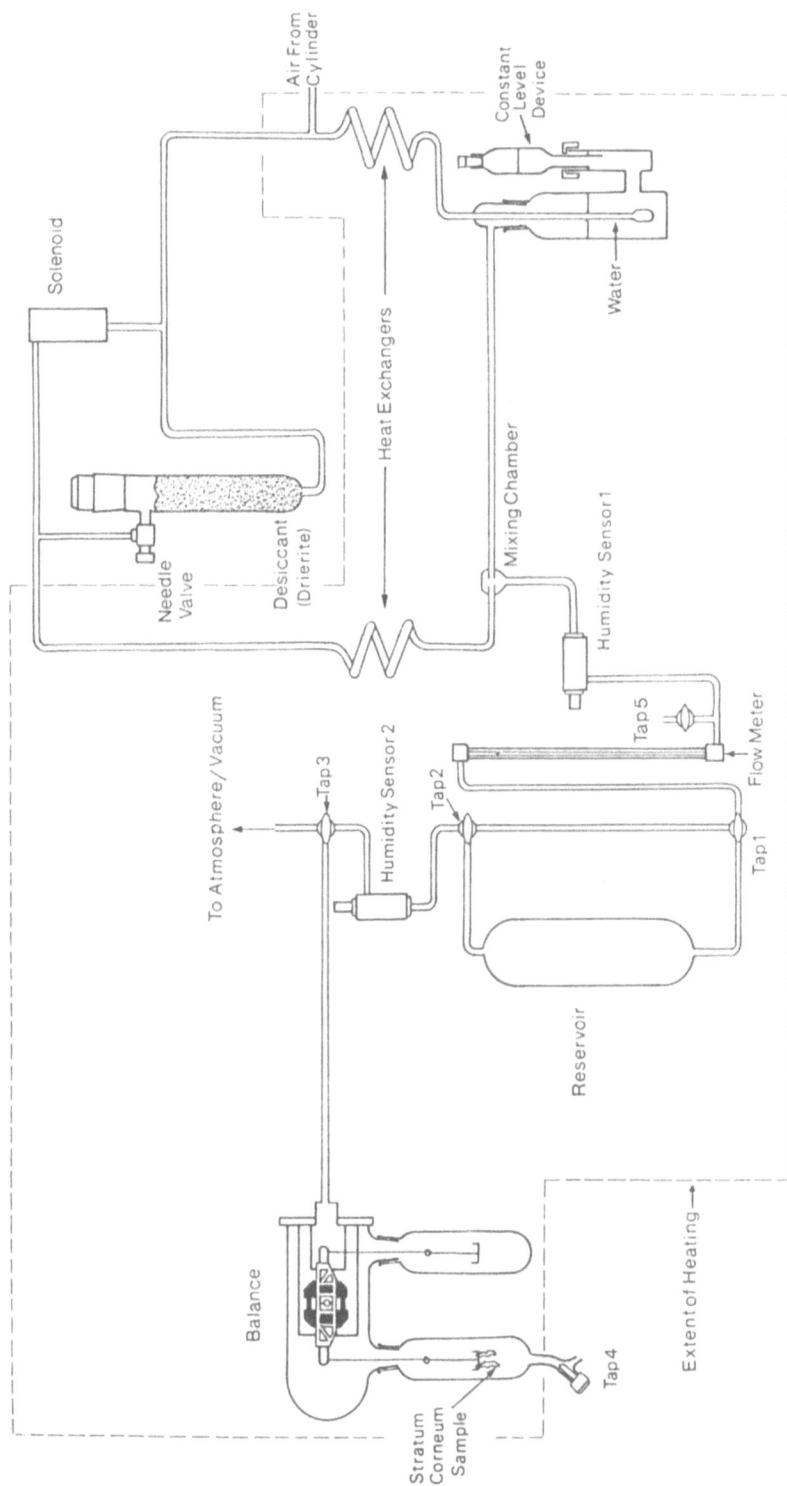

Figure 12.1 Apparatus for water vapour sorption and desorption studies in a stratum corneum in vitro. The dotted lines indicate the equipment housed in a controlled temperature cabinet at $32 \pm 0.2°C$

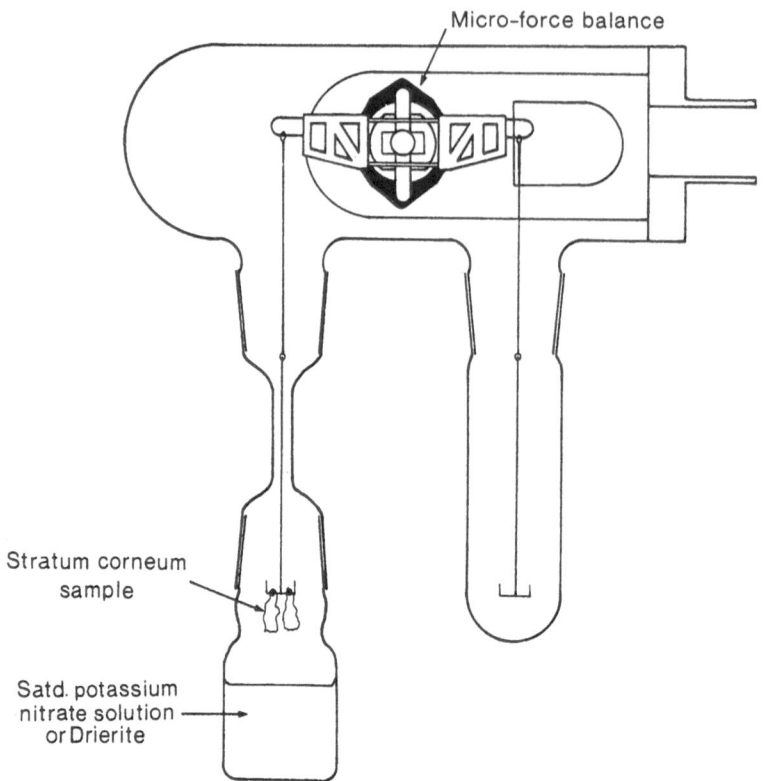

Figure 12.2 Modification of the apparatus microbalance chamber for the stationary experiments

Treatment of the stratum corneum samples

Pieces of stratum corneum were treated in the following manner:

(1) Untreated skin, washed in distilled water.

(2) Stratum corneum soaked in 5 ml of 12% w/v sodium chloride solution for 12 hours.

(3) Stratum corneum soaked in 5 ml of 12% w/v urea solution for 12 hours.

(4) Stratum corneum soaked in 5 ml of 12% w/v urea and sodium chloride solution for 12 hours.

All samples were washed briefly in distilled water prior to testing on the flow and stationary system or diffusion cell apparatus.

It has been established since the 1940s that urea and sodium chloride are of benefit in the treatment of various dry skin conditions[16]. Swanbeck[17] published a patent in which he claimed that a combination of urea and sodium chloride produces a synergistic water-retaining effect compared to either treatment alone. Frithz[18] claimed similar results using 4% urea and 4% sodium chloride in in vivo subjective tests. Other authors, however, who used 12% urea and 12% sodium chloride combination disagreed[19]. This present study was initiated in order to investigate the claim by Swanbeck of synergism in the water-retaining effect of urea and sodium chloride combinations. We found (Table 12.1) that both urea and sodium chloride increased the water content of the stratum corneum samples by approximately 2-fold. However, the 12% urea and 12% sodium chloride combination was not significantly different ($p > 0.05$) to either of these treatments alone.

Table 12.1 Ratio increases or decreases in water vapour uptake (treated:untreated control) after 24 hours for one stratum corneum sample. There was no significant difference ($p > 0.05$) between treatments

Skin treatment	Relative humidity %	
	0-91	91-0
Stationary system		
NaCl (12% w/v)	1.2	1.5
Urea (12% w/v)	1.4	1.6
NaCl + Urea	2.2	2.3
Flow system		
NaCl (12% w/v)	1.3	1.2
Urea (12% w/v)	3.3	3.0
NaCl + Urea	3.2	3.2

An interesting observation which emerged from these experiments was that a significant difference could be seen with sorption and desorption patterns between the stationary (S) and flow (F) systems (Figure 12.3, Table 12.2). At 24 hours in the S system the water vapour was still being sorbed, whilst in the F system the stratum corneum samples had already reached an equilibrium water content. This pattern was observed in over 200 experiments performed and for some runs in which we tested for 3-4 days the S samples had not reached equilibrium by the end of the experiment. Anderson et al.[14] reported similar sorption and desorption patterns with their stationary system and found that equilibrium water contents were reached only after 14 days. There was no significant difference ($p > 0.05$) between the initial absorption diffusion coefficients (Table 12.2) of F and S systems or treated and untreated stratum corneum samples. However, the initial desorption coefficients were always higher in the S system. The difference may be accounted for by the fact that in the S system the final water content was higher than in the F system and when the sample then came into contact

107

with dry air, the excess moisture was lost more readily from the S sample. Most authors[8] agreed with the observation that desorption was a faster process than sorption.

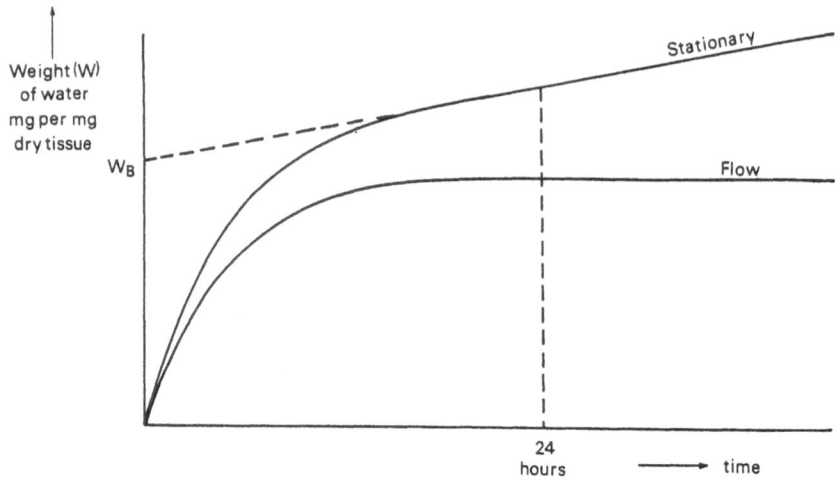

Figure 12.3 An example of a plot of weight of water vapour sorbed (W) per mg of dry tissue against time in hours

Table 12.2 Values (W) of water vapour sorbed or desorbed in 24 hours per mg of dry stratum corneum and initial diffusion coefficients (D_i) x 10^{-7} cm^2 h^{-1} for untreated and treated stratum corneum samples taken from a female, aged 74

Skin treatment	Flow (F) or stationary (S) system	Relative humidity %			
		0-91		91-0	
		W	D_i	W	D_i
Controls	F	0.0649	2.31	0.0617	5.41
	S	0.121	0.91	0.112	11.9
NaCl 12% w/v for 12 hours	F	0.0825	1.47	0.0730	6.15
	S	0.141	0.60	0.166	18.6
Urea 12% w/v for 12 hours	F	0.216	0.55	0.186	8.50
	S	0.172	0.37	0.176	7.16
Urea 12% + NaCl 12% w/v for 12 hours	F	0.208	0.26	0.198	0.87
	S	0.261	0.30	0.252	7.46

Anderson et al.[14] proposed that there are at least three types of water within the hydrated stratum corneum. The first species is 'strongly bound' water probably associated with the polar groups of the keratin side-chains in the corneocytes. Hydration kinetic data suggest that this initially 'bound' water increases as the total water content rises (i.e as the water activity of the environment increases). These authors' data for desorption using disrupted tissue samples and a nuclear magnetic resonance technique suggests that this water is mainly intracellular. This 'strongly bound' water can be subdivided into two fractions: primary hydration of ionic groups and the associated secondary hydration. The third water species is present at higher humidity levels and is more like bulk water in its hydrogen-bonding capabilities. This 'free' water is not strongly associated with the stratum corneum constituents and is present intercellularly. The ability of the stratum corneum to retain liquid water either as a surface film or within intercellular spaces has been shown to depend upon the presence of skin lipids[20]. We postulate that in our system the passage of air prevented the formation of this third water species and only the 'bound' type of water was present in the stratum corneum samples. In the S system, hydration swelled the corneum membrane, intercellular channels containing liquid water formed and the water then slowly diffused into the corneocyte.

In skin in vivo there are naturally occurring hygroscopic substances which aid the water-retaining capacity of the stratum corneum. Among these are urea and sodium chloride which are provided by eccrine sweat. These substances disrupt the protein matrix owing to their location between protein chain segments and lead to increased hydration. Hence in skin from older patients (as was used in these experiments) addition of sodium chloride or urea to stratum corneum, which is already depleted of these substances, may lead to an increased water-retaining capacity of the skin.

DIFFUSION CELL METHOD

Stratum corneum samples were prepared as reported previously, and mounted in glass diffusion cells (Figure 12.4) similar to those used by Blank et al.[12]. 1 ml of saturated potassium nitrate solution (kept at 32 ± 0.5°C) was placed in both donor and receptor sides of the cell and all the cells were placed in a water bath at 32 ± 0.5°C to equilibrate for 3 days. Only the vapour above the solution at a relative humidity of 91% contacted the stratum corneum, and in addition magnetic stirrers were placed in each side of the cell. The cell itself was sealed around the stratum corneum sample with paraffin wax. 10 µl of undiluted tritiated water (HTO) was then added to the potassium nitrate solution on the donor side, allowed to mix and then a 100 µl sample was taken and placed in 5 ml of scintillation fluid (Optiphase Safe, LKB). All samples removed were replaced by an equal volume of saturated potassium nitrate solution. Two 100 µl samples were also taken from the receptor side of two cells chosen at random to act as initial blank checks. All samples were counted for 10 minutes in a Packard Tricarb 460C scintillation counter. The donor side gave counts of 45-50 million counts in 10 minutes. Subsequently 100 µl samples of the receptor side were taken at 1 hourly intervals for 10 hours beginning 24 hours after the initial HTO injection. A period of 24 hours was allowed for the cells to reach steady state, a value derived from our experimental data. When sampling was complete the cells were washed five times with distilled water and then completely filled with one of the following:

(1) 12% w/v sodium chloride solution for 12 hours,

(2) 12% w/v urea solution for 12 hours,

(3) 12% w/v urea + 12% sodium chloride solution for 12 hours.

The solutions were then discarded and the cells were washed once with distilled water and left for 6 hours in a desiccator. The sampling experiment was then repeated.

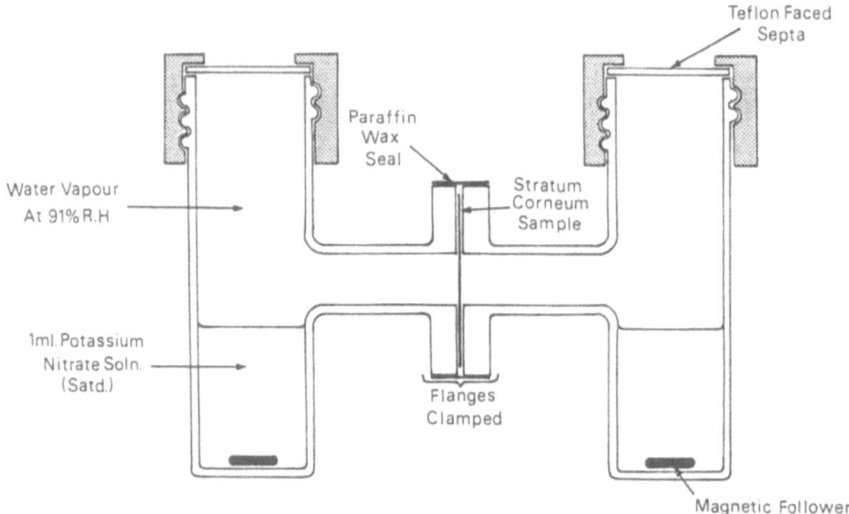

Figure 12.4 A glass diffusion cell for vapour transport measurements

A control HTO run was followed by a treatment run which in turn was followed by a control rerun experiment. The stratum corneum pieces were then replaced and the entire experiment was repeated with a new treatment. An example of results obtained from one piece of autopsied skin sample is given in Table 12.3.

Damage ratios (DR) of values greater than one suggest that some change has occurred in the stratum corneum sample either by the treatment or the washout procedure. The results of one skin sample (Table 12.3) show that both urea and sodium chloride increased the water vapour penetration and that the sodium chloride and urea combination produced a statistically significant increase in the effect observed. However, another skin sample tested did not

Table 12.3 Permeability coefficients (k_p) x 10^{-4} cm h^{-1} and standard deviations from the mean (SD) for one (treated and control) stratum corneum sample. The samples were changed between runs 1 and 2 and 2 and 3. DR is Damage Ratio (see text)

Run no.	Treatment	No. of Experiments	Mean k_p x 10^{-4} cm h^{-1} ± SD	DR
1	Control	9	8.7 ± 3.7	-
	NaCl 12%	8	12.1 ± 5.6	-
	Control rerun	8	14.6 ± 8.2	1.7
2	Control	7	11.1 ± 6.6	-
	Urea 12%	7	47.6 ± 17.9	-
	Control rerun	6	59.1 ± 33.0	5.3
3	Control	8	13.9 ± 6.2	-
	NaCl 12% + urea 12%	7	46.3 ± 8.7	-
	Control rerun	5	48.6 ± 10.2	3.5

produce this significant increase. The damage ratio was always higher following urea treatment alone or the sodium chloride and urea combination treatment. These results were expected since urea is known to be a proteolytic agent at the concentrations used[22].

ACKNOWLEDGEMENTS

The authors are grateful to Pharmacia AB, Sweden for financial assistance for the support of a postdoctoral fellow (B.B.M.-M.) and to Mr I. L. Waller and Mrs P.C. Rowland for their technical assistance.

REFERENCES

1. Scheuplein, R.J. and Blank, I.H. (1971). Permeability of the skin. Physiol. Rev., **51**, 702-47
2. Middleton, J.D. and Allen, B.M. (1973). The influence of temperature and humidity on stratum corneum and its relation to skin chapping. J. Soc. Cosm. Chem., **24**, 239-43
3. Blank, I.H. (1952). Factors which influence the water content of the stratum corneum. J. Invest. Dermatol., **18**, 433-40
4. Flesch, P. and Escoda, E.C.J. (1957). Deficient water-binding in pathologic horny layers. J. Invest. Dermatol., **28**, 5-13
5. Grice, K.A. and Bettley, F.A. (1967). Skin water loss and accidental hypothermia in psoriasis, ichthyosis, and erythroderma. Br. Med. J., **4**, 195-8
6. Frost, P., Weinstein, G.D., Bothwell, J.W. and Wildnauser, R. (1968). Ichthyosiform dermatoses. III. Studies of transepidermal water loss. Arch. Dermatol., **98**, 230-3
7. Jacobi, O.K. (1959). About the mechanism of moisture regulation in the horny layer of the skin. Proc. Sci. Sect. Toilet Goods Assoc., **31**, 22-30
8. Scheuplein, R.J. and Morgan, L.J. (1967). 'Bound water' in keratin membranes measured by a microbalance technique. Nature (London), **214**, 456-8
9. Scheuplein, R.J. (1980). Percutaneous absorption theoretical aspects. In Mauvais-Jarvis, P., Vickers, C.F.H. and Wepierre, J. (eds.) Percutaneous Absorption of Steroids. pp 12-13. (London: Academic Press)
10. Wurster, D.E. and Kramer, S.F. (1961). Investigations of some factors influencing percutaneous absorption. J. Pharm. Sci., **50**, 288-93
11. Fritsch, W.F. and Stoughton, R.B. (1963). The effect of temperature and humidity on the penetration of ^{14}C acetylsalicylic acid in excised human skin. J. Invest. Dermatol., **41**, 307-10
12. Fick, A. (1855). Uber diffusion. Poggendorffs. Ann., **94**, 59-86

13. Flynn, G.L. (1979). Topical drug absorption and topical pharmaceutical systems. In Banker, G.S. and Rhodes, C.T. (eds.) Modern Pharmaceutics (Drugs and the Pharmaceutical Sciences). Chap. 8, pp 263-325. (London: Dekker)
14. Anderson, R.L., Cassidy, J.M., Hansen, J.R. and Yellin, W. (1973). Hydration of stratum corneum. Biopolymers, 12, 2789-802
15. Kligman, A.M. and Christophers, E. (1963). Preparation of isolated sheets of human stratum corneum. Arch. Dermatol., 88, 702-5
16. Rattner, H. (1943). Use of urea in hand creams. Arch. Dermatol., 48, 47-51
17. Swanbeck, G. (1975). U.K. Patent No. 1411432
18. Frithz, A. (1983). Investigation of Cortesal, a hydrocortisone cream and its water-retaining cream base in the treatment of xerotic skin and dry eczemas. Curr. Ther. Res., 33, 930-5
19. Gip, L. and Lundberg, M.A. (1985). A double-blind trial of a new psoriatic cream containing urea and sodium chloride. Curr. Ther. Res., 37, 797-804
20. Foreman, M.I., Bladon, P. and Pelling, P. (1979). Proton NMR studies of human stratum corneum. Bioeng. Skin, 2, 48-58
21. Blank, I.H., Moloney, J., Emslie, A.G., Simon, I. and Apt, C. (1984). The diffusion of water across the stratum corneum as a function of its water content. J. Invest. Dermatol., 82, 188-94
22. Swanbeck, G. and Rajka, G. (1970). Antipruritic effect of urea solution. Acta Dermatol., 50, 225-8

Section IV

CHANNELS OF COMMUNICATION IN SKIN

Chapter 13

Measurement of cutaneous blood flow

P A Payne

INTRODUCTION

The measurement of skin blood flow is an activity that has been pursued for many years. However, in the last decade or so there appears to be a significant number of advances in the technology of skin blood flow measurement.

In the preface to the Proceedings of a Conference on Skin Blood Flow Measurement[1], the statement is made that 'measurement of volume blood flow through the skin is not difficult, but that the measurement of the distribution of this volume flow through the various interrelated segments which make up the skin's micro-vasculature is a difficult and probably unsolved problem'. A most important aspect of skin blood flow is that associated with nutrition and it is known that the nutritional flow through the skin is often far less than the total skin blood flow. The reasons for this have been investigated and have to do with the role that skin blood flow plays in the thermoregulation of the body, plus, to a lesser extent, the involvement of skin blood flow in the control of blood pressure.

The measurement of nutritional blood flow in the skin is a difficult problem, as mentioned previously, and requires a measurement technique that can identify the flow within the nutritional capillaries and isolate that flow component from the very complex flow regimes that exist in other regions of the skin.

In this chapter, a brief review of the anatomy and physiology of the vasculature of the skin is provided, followed by a review of various methods of measuring skin blood flow. As already stated, the most important measurement associated with skin blood flow is one that will give rise to estimations of nutrient flow and a technique capable of making such a measurement is presented later in this chapter.

ANATOMY AND PHYSIOLOGY OF THE VASCULATURE OF THE SKIN

The blood vessels within the skin are extremely varied in terms of diameter, wall thickness and the direction in which they run with respect to the skin surface. Figure 13.1 provides a diagrammatic view of the various blood vessels referred to and in terms of nutritional flow, the papillary capillaries are of most significance. It is the flow within these blood vessels that provides the necessary nutrition for the cell differentiation that occurs in the basal

115

membrane of the epidermis. This process is the renewal process that compensates for the continual loss of the outer cells of the stratum corneum. These vessels are very thin walled and consist of single layers of endothelial cells supported by a basement membrane. Their structure and function is optimized to enable the necessary exchange of material between the red blood cells and the surrounding tissue. Indeed, in passing down a capillary, a red blood cell is forced to deform to a very large degree, which presumably also assists in the process of exchange of materials.

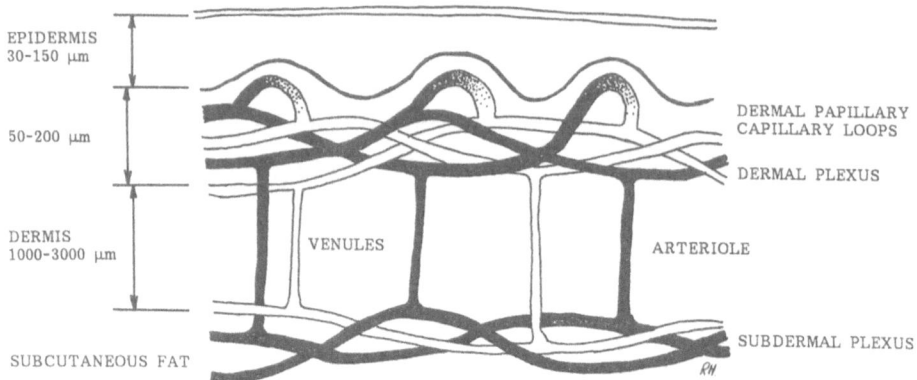

Figure 13.1 The microanatomy of skin and the microcirculation. Dimensions shown are approximate

MEASUREMENT METHODS

As mentioned before, there are numerous methods that have been devised to enable skin blood flow measurements to be undertaken. In some cases these have been employed in order to obtain an understanding of normal skin blood flow and in others the techniques have been applied in studies relating to numerous disease processes that affect the flow of blood in the skin. The techniques available are listed below with a brief description of each one.

Light microscopy[2]

The papillary capillaries can be clearly seen through the surface of the skin using a stereo microscope. Workers using this technique have used materials such as liquid paraffin or clear nail varnish to optically clarify the upper layers of the skin in order to improve this visibility. They also report that lower blood vessels of the skin circulation are visible, but with some difficulty. The technique allows only a subjective judgement of skin blood flow changes, but has proved useful in one study undertaken to understand the effect of the use of a heated probe during transcutaneous pO_2 measurements.

Nail bed microscopy[3]

The capillaries in the region of the nail fold are particularly amenable to observation via a light microscope. This is primarily because they tend to run more parallel to the skin surface than elsewhere. By linking the microscope to a television and video recorder system, it is possible to study the movement of red blood cells through the capillaries and by use of the recorder replaying at slow speeds, estimates of red blood cell velocities through the capillaries can be made. In addition, individual capillaries can be subjected to a pressure measurement technique[4] providing additional important information. The skin is again treated with liquid paraffin wax or clear nail varnish to aid in the visualization of the capillaries.

Infra-red thermography[5]

The use of a thermographic technique to track changes in flow which in turn cause changes in skin temperature has been described by numerous authors. In terms of blood flow measurement the technique is subjective. Its major advantages are that it is non-invasive and that it acquires information from large areas of the skin, in contrast to most other techniques which are, in effect, point measurements.

Microwave thermography[6]

A system using a 10 GHz microwave thermograph has been employed to examine the effects of peripheral vascular disease. Although described in relationship to skin blood flow, the technique is really more associated with the assessment of tissue perfusion down to depths of up to 3 cm below the skin surface. The technique is related to the infra-red thermography technique in that it also detects electromagnetic radiation, but at a different region of the spectrum.

Thermal conductance[7]

This is probably the oldest of the skin blood flow measurement techniques and relies on placing a small heated disc upon the skin surface, the temperature of which is about 3°C above the temperature of an outer annulus within which thermocouples are placed to monitor temperature changes. These changes will occur due to the alteration in thermal conductance of the skin between the disc and the annulus as the skin blood flow alters. The difficulty associated with the technique is that for a given geometry of the device, the assumption of a particular skin thickness has to be made in order to obtain information. It is known, however, that epidermis and dermis dimensions change markedly around the body and, in addition, are greatly altered from one subject to another. It has, nevertheless, proved a useful and effective measurement technique.

Photoreflectance plethysmography[8]

This again is one of the very early techniques that have been used to investigate peripheral circulation, although it was not until advances in semiconductor technology occurred, that direct applications to skin blood flow could be investigated. In the case of skin blood flow, the normal method is to apply a source and detector adjacent to one another on the surface of the skin. Light wavelengths of between 800 and 1200 nm have been employed and these appear to correspond to a depth of penetration in human skin of between 1.2 and 2.0 mm. Such wavelengths are conveniently produced by light emitting diodes. The photodetector must obviously be selected to have a spectral response that is in accordance with the source and the results obtained contain both a pulsatile component which is in phase with the cardiac cycle, together with a component at a much lower frequency. The lower frequency component may well be associated with the control mechanisms that vary the overall blood flow in the skin. The data obtained from such measurements are only a relative measurement of skin blood flow.

Isotope clearance techniques[9]

A number of isotopes have been employed to measure skin blood flow using standard methods of counting the particles emitted following introduction into the dermis. Early work used radioactive sodium and the subsequent use of radioactive xenon became a more popular technique. However, there are problems with xenon due to its lipophilic properties and sodium is difficult to work with because of the rather short half-life. These problems have led to investigations of technetium as a suitable isotope and this appears to have considerable advantages. The major disadvantage associated with isotope clearance techniques is that the isotopes themselves must be introduced into the skin using a suitable hypodermic syringe and, in addition to the difficulties of doing this in diseased skin regions, there is the added possibility that the reaction produced by the superficial injury inevitably involved is likely to change the pattern of skin blood flow.

Fluorescence techniques[10]

In this method, an intravenous injection of sodium fluorescein is followed by measurement of the fluorescence of the material, whilst the diffusion processes across capillary membranes reduce the effect. It is thus claimed to be a method of measuring capillary blood flow. Some workers use a slow intravenous infusion rather than a bolus dose in order to reduce histamine release-related side-effects. Again, the major disadvantage of this technique would appear to be the difficulties of performing a measurement of this nature at wound sites and also the effects of the bolus injection of infusion.

Laser doppler techniques[11-13]

These techniques have probably become the most popular methods for measuring skin blood flow and have found wide application in the assessment of burns, the monitoring of the results of plastic surgery and studies of blood flow in Raynaud's disease.

The technique relies upon the well-known Doppler effect, in which light of a given frequency which is scattered off a moving particle such as a red blood cell is changed in frequency, dependent on the velocity of the particle. The technique relies upon the coherence properties of laser light and has been shown to be capable of detecting velocities down to 0.007 m s^{-1}. The processing of the signals from a laser Doppler flowmeter differ between different commercial instruments, but the most common approach is the use of weighted estimates of the bandwidth of the electrical signal obtained. It is the form of weighting that appears to differ mostly and it is not entirely clear whether the signal obtained is linearly related to flow. The best that has been accomplished so far is to show that the technique correlates well with other more traditional methods.

The penetration of the laser light will depend to some extent upon the power used and to a large extent, upon the wavelength. Comments in the literature indicate that it is believed that the penetration is anything from 0.3 mm to some 1.5 mm. In the context of papillary capillary flow measurements, then 0.3 mm would be acceptable, but anything much greater than this is bound to include the effects of flow in other vessels within the skin.

Pulsed doppler ultrasound[14]

Doppler ultrasound is a widely used technique for the measurement of blood flow in deep vessels within the body. It has the advantages of being both non-invasive and relatively inexpensive. The more recent use of pulsed Doppler ultrasound has enabled the study of the velocity profiles within the major blood vessels and has enabled, in addition, the non-invasive measurement of absolute blood flow by combining this measurement with one which obtains data on the diameter of the lumen.

It is a fairly natural extension to consider using this technique for skin blood flow. In this context, the major advantage is that very accurate control over the depth from which measurements are taken is possible by the use of range gating. Further details on the instrumentation and applications of this method are provided in the next section.

PULSED DOPPLER SKIN BLOOD FLOWMETER

Although the laser Doppler technique uses a similar physical basis for its operation, the ability to range gate such a system does not exist because of the very high propagation velocity of electromagnetic radiation through the skin. In order to accomplish a range gated approach using the laser Doppler system, switching times of a few picoseconds would be required to modulate the laser energy. The advantage of turning to an interrogating energy such as ultrasound is that its propagation velocity is much lower (a factor of 2×10^5 approximately). Thus, in order to range gate for the necessary period, we are dealing with a gating time of approximately 1.0-1.5 µs. This ensures that we achieve a sample volume of a size to enclose, for example, the papillary capillaries and at the same time exclude the influence of other vessels.

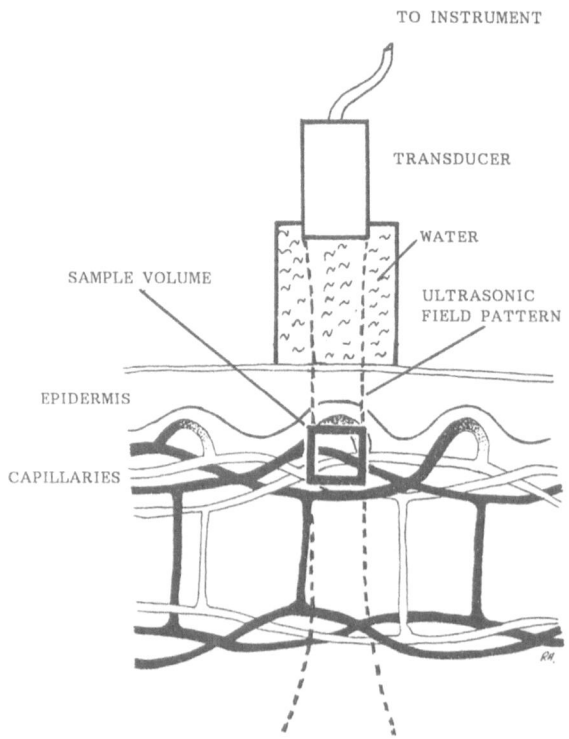

TO INSTRUMENT

TRANSDUCER

WATER

SAMPLE VOLUME

ULTRASONIC
FIELD PATTERN

EPIDERMIS

CAPILLARIES

Figure 13.2 Method of examining capillary blood flow using pulsed Doppler ultrasound and thus defining a sample volume

Figure 13.2 shows diagrammatically the way in which the system operates. A brief tone burst of 1.0-1.5 μs in length at an accurately controlled ultrasound frequency (somewhere between 20 and 40 MHz has been found acceptable) is emitted by the transducer. This tone burst of ultrasound travels through a water bath until it strikes the stratum corneum. At this point, some of the energy is reflected back towards the transducer and some will continue on. The same effect will occur as the pulse of ultrasound travels down through the skin and encounters layers within the skin such as that between the dermis and the subcutaneous tissue. However, in addition to these reflections, the other effect that occurs is concerned with the red blood cells that are moving in the various parts of the vasculature. Providing the wavelength of the ultrasound energy is large compared with the diameter of the red blood cells, then Rayleigh scattering will occur. This has the effect of returning some of the incident energy to the transducer, but at a slightly shifted frequency dependent on the Doppler effect. The frequency shift is readily measured and is related to the velocity of the red blood cell involved. Clearly, there is an angular consideration to take into account. However, since the papillary capillaries run almost vertically with respect to the skin surface on many regions of interest, then any error due to the non-normal aspect of the blood flow is much reduced. A major feature of the instrument is the ability to move the sample volume to any position within the skin and to vary its length, thus providing a measurement for any of the flow regimes.

Analysis of the Doppler signal frequency spectrum

The red blood cells travelling through the capillaries are known[15] to have velocities distributed over a range of something like 0-0.6 mm s^{-1}. This is somewhat variable and the variability arises because red blood cells seem to move through the capillaries in a rather erratic manner as observed using the light microscope techniques referred to earlier. The effect of this is to produce a range of Doppler shifts and, therefore, a range of frequencies associated with the Doppler signal. In communications engineering terms, this is referred to as a frequency spectrum and there are numerous ways of analysing such a signal. In the case of the skin flowmeter, it has been convenient to plot these spectra graphically and to obtain flow data from these plots. A typical normal skin blood flow spectrum is shown in Figure 13.3, where the horizontal scale is calibrated in both frequency shift and velocity associated with such a shift. The vertical scale represents the strength of the signal at any one of the shift frequencies and may be related to the number of red blood cells that are moving at that particular velocity. Thus, if we wish to compute the total flow that has been interrogated by the ultrasound beam, we merely need to take the area under the graph. However, this assumes that the instrument behaves in a linear manner with respect to changes in flow. A calibration exercise is therefore essential to establish this.

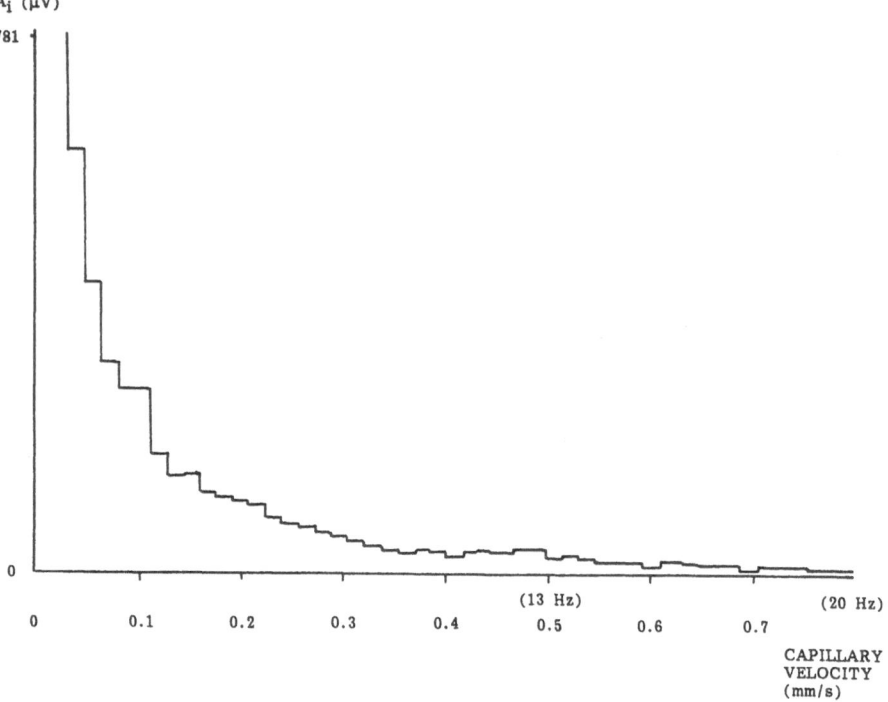

Figure 13.3 Normal capillary blood flow

Calibration of the skin blood flow instrument

A flow rig was constructed which enabled accurate determinations of the flow of milk, which has suitable scattering properties, to be determined. The milk was allowed to pass through a narrow bore, thin wall silicone-rubber tube and the ultrasound transducer was adjusted so that it obtained scattered signals from the milk flowing through the tube. In Figure 13.4, three spectra are shown for three separate flow rates through the silicone tubing and in Figure 13.5, the area under each of the three spectra are plotted against the accurately determined flow rate obtained by collecting the milk from the flow rig in a calibrated cylinder. As can be seen, the results provide evidence of good linear response over flow rates between 1.5 and 3.8 μl s^{-1}. These may be related to the estimated flow in units of microvolt-Hertz by the slope of the calibration line, and the calibration factor for the instrument of 1 μV Hz is equivalent to 5.5 nl s^{-1}. However, the resolution for the data obtained, in which the vertical scale is 488 μV full scale, is no better than 5 μV Hz corresponding to a flow rate of 28 nl s^{-1}. A further factor that must be considered in looking at the lower limit of resolution for the instrument is the inherent noise and, from previous experiments, this has been shown to be typically less than 10 μV over the frequency range considered.

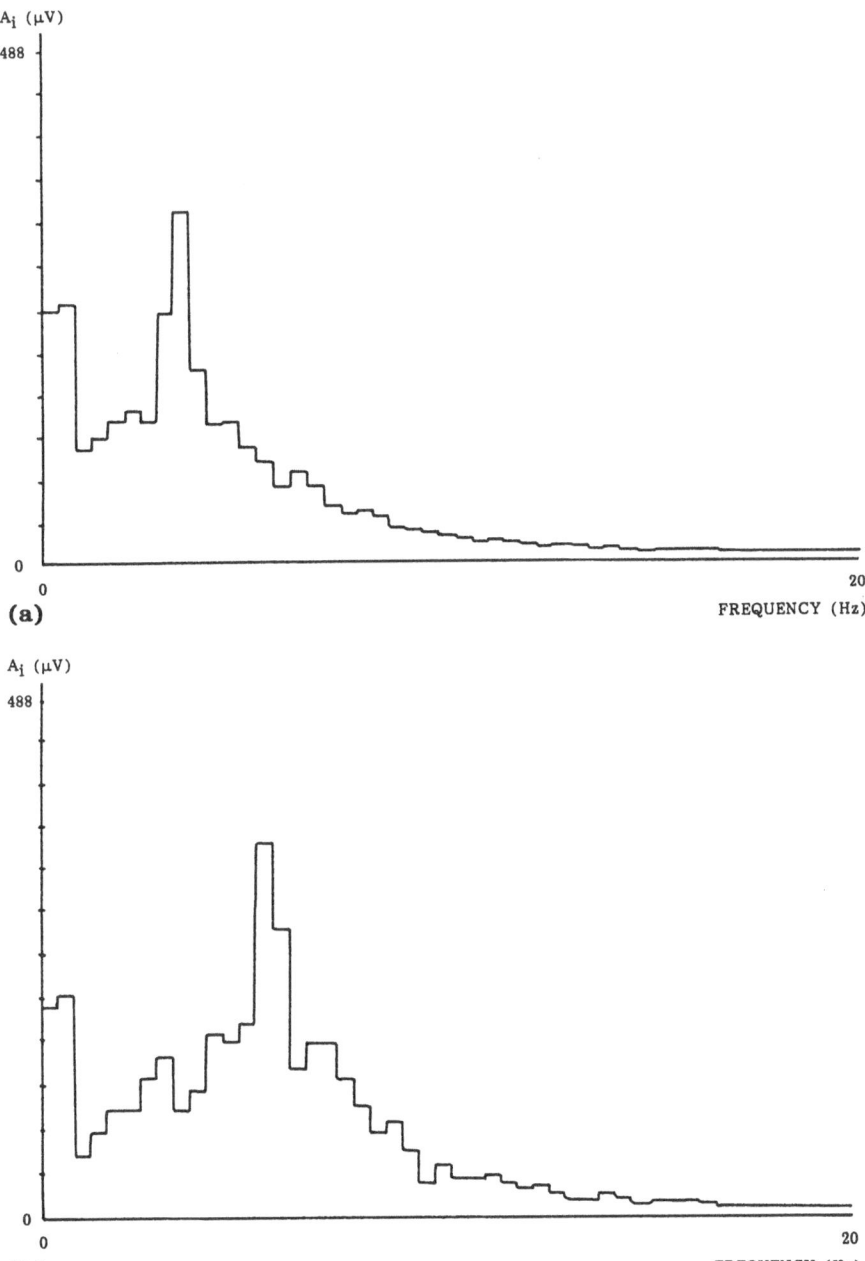

Figure 13.4   Calibration data for the pulsed Doppler flowmeter:
(a) 1650 nl s^{-1} (flow measured using calibrated cylinder)
(b) 2300 nl s^{-1} (flow measured using calibrated cylinder)
(c) 3670 nl s^{-1} (flow measured using calibrated cylinder)

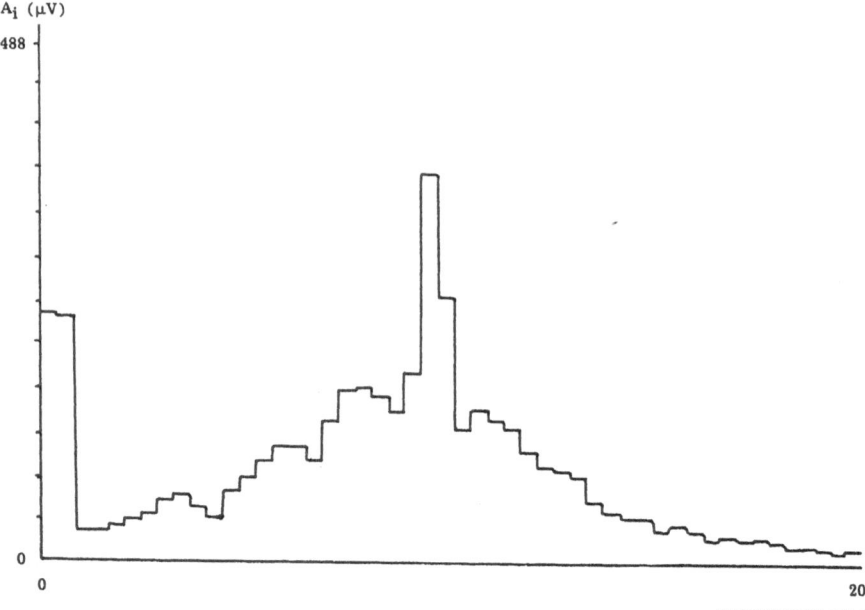

Figure 13.4 (c)

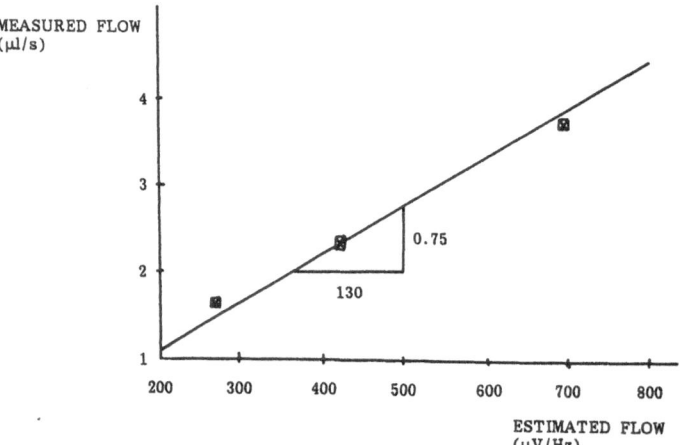

Figure 13.5 Data from Figure 13.4 plotted against measured flow to give a calibration constant for instrument of 0.0055 μl s^{-1}

Absolute measurement of skin blood flow

The ability to determine flow, rather than simply velocity as in the case of most techniques, is in part due to the calibration graph referred to earlier, but is also due to the fact that for a given ultrasound transducer, we can determine fairly accurately the shape of the effective transmitter beam, as well as the shape of the receiver field. Thus, we can consider the transducer to interrogate a known volume of skin tissue (the sample volume). This means that the flow measurement obtained is a flow measurement for a known volume of tissue which will be measured in units of litres per metre^3 per second ($1 m^{-3} s^{-1}$).

For the normal skin blood flow shown in Figure 13.3, the flow was equivalent to 220 μV Hz. Using the calibration factor for the instrument, this turns out to be a flow rate of 1.2 $\mu l s^{-1}$. Knowing the characteristics of the ultrasound transducer used enabled a calculation of blood flow per tissue volume and per tissue area. The latter figure turned out to be 15 $\mu l m^{-2} s^{-1}$)which is in good agreement with published data (12 to 60 $\mu l m^{-2} s^{-1}$)[16].

Examples of flowmeter measurements under conditions of altered skin blood flow

Figure 13.6 shows the effects of changing the skin blood flow in a normal subject due first to heating the skin and secondly, to the effects of cigarette smoking. The response of the instrument to a variety of other stimuli such as exercise, cold, the Valsalva manoeuvre, and the raising and lowering of the arm, in the case of flow measurements carried out on the forearm or the digits have all demonstrated the effectiveness of the device.

CONCLUSIONS

There is a growing clinical interest in development of techniques for the measurement of skin blood flow. Numerous techniques have been developed over the years and many of these have been used to good effect in development and understanding of the flow of blood in the skin. However, methods that are of use in a research environment are very often inapplicable clinically. The recent interest in the use of laser Doppler techniques arises primarily from the fact that it is a convenient and relatively simple technique to employ, which lends itself to the clinical environment.

As this chapter has pointed out, there are limitations to the use of the laser Doppler method and these arise primarily from the lack of control over the laser light penetration. An alternative method is to employ the ultrasound technique that has been described and this shows great promise for future research and clinical applications.

125

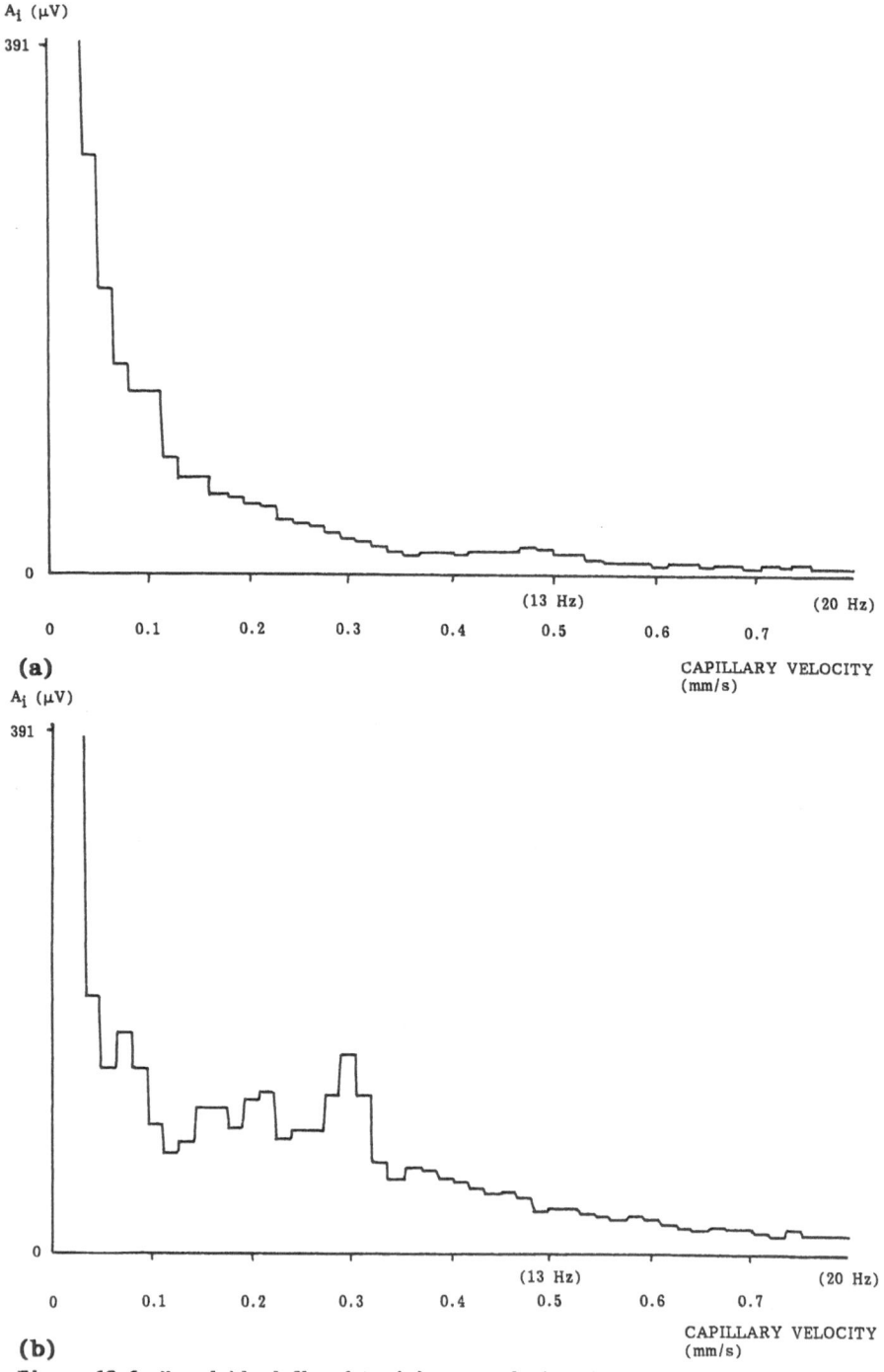

Figure 13.6 Normal blood flow data **(a)** compared with the effect due to cigarette smoking **(b)** and to heating the skin **(c)**

126

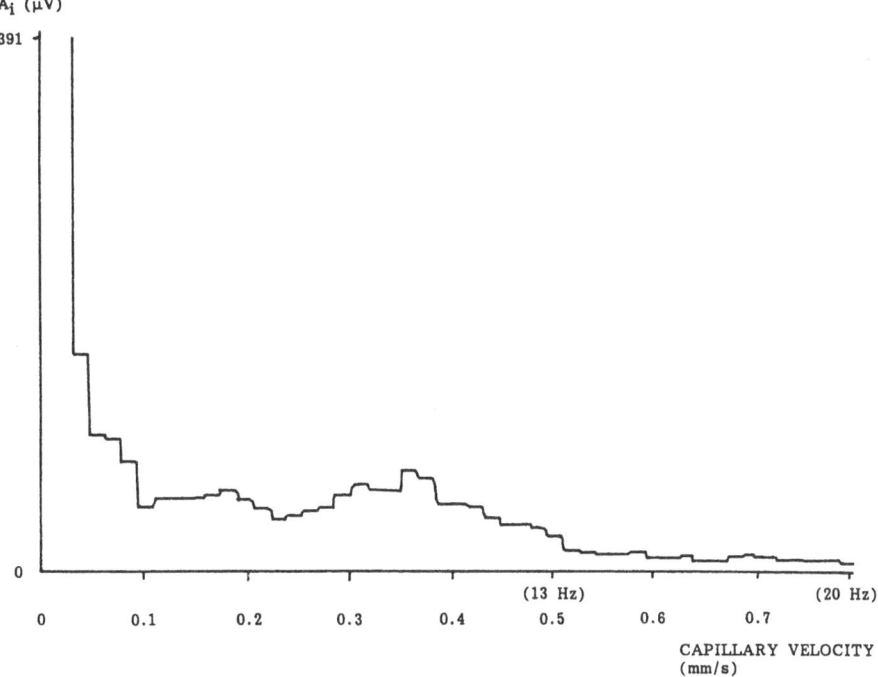

Figure 13.6 (c)

ACKNOWLEDGEMENTS

Work on pulsed Doppler ultrasound measurements of skin blood flow was supported by SERC and Hoffmann La Roche. Contributions were made by members of the Ultrasound Research Group of the Department of Instrumentation and Analytical Science, UMIST, and the author records his thanks to past and present members of the Group.

REFERENCES

1. Spence, V.A. and Sheldon, C.D. (eds.) (1985). Practical Aspects of Skin Blood Flow Measurements. BES Conference Proceedings, Vol.1. (London: Biological Engineering Society)
2. Shakespeare, P.G. and Swain, I.D. (1985). Skin blood flow and $TcpO_2$ measurement. In Spence, V.A. and Sheldon, C.D. (eds.) Practical Aspects of Skin Blood Flow Measurements. pp 78-81. (London: Biological Engineering Society)
3. Fagrell, B., Frohnek, A. and Butaliatta, M. (1977). A microscope television system for studying flow velocity in human skin capillaries. Am. J. Physiol., **233**(2), H318-21
4. Tooke, J.E. and Rayman, G. (1985). The investigation of foot skin microcirculation in diabetes mellitus. In Spence, V.A. and Sheldon, C.D. (eds.) Practical Aspects of Skin Blood Flow Measurements. pp 73-7. (London: Biological Engineering Society)
5. Ring, E.F.J. (1986). Skin temperature measurement. Bioeng. Skin, **2**, 15-30
6. Monson, J.R.T., Abd-Alrazzak, M.M., Ausobsky, J., Matthews, P.A. and Kester, R.C. (1985). The use of microwave emission thermography in peripheral vascular disease - a preliminary study. In Spence, V.A. and Sheldon, C.D. (eds.) Practical Aspects of Skin Blood Flow Measurements. pp 69-72. (London: Biological Engineering Society)

7. Payne, P.A. (1984). Measurement of skin blood flow. Electronics and Power, **30**, 219-21

8. Mani, R. and White, J.E. (1985). The use of photoreflectance probes and transcutaneous oxygen electrodes for investigation of leg ulcers. Bioeng. Skin, **1**, 207-17

9. McCollum, P.T., Spence, V.A., Walker, W.F., Murdoch, G., Swanson, A.J.G. and Turner, M.S. (1985). Antipyrine clearance from the skin of the foot and the lower leg in critical ischaemia: clinical implications. In Spence, V.A. and Sheldon, C.D. (eds.) Practical Aspects of Skin Blood Flow Measurements. pp 47-51. (London: Biological Engineering Society)

10. Silverman, D.G., Cedrone, F.A. and Hurford, W.E. (1981). Monitoring tissue elimination of fluorescein with the perfusion fluorometer: a new method to assess capillary blood flow. Surgery, **89**, 409

11. Fairs, S.L.E., De Trafford, J.C. and Roberts, V.C. (1985). Optical methods for measuring blood flow in skin. In Spence, V.A. and Sheldon, C.D. (eds.) Practical Aspects of Skin Blood Flow. pp 11-17. (London: Biological Engineering Society)

12. Almond, N.E., Jones, D.P., Bowcock, S.A. and Cooke, E.D. (1985). A laser Doppler blood flowmeter used to detect thermal entrainment in normal persons and patients with Raynaud's phenomenon. In Spence, V.A. and Sheldon, C.D. (eds.) Practical Aspects of Skin Blood Flow. pp 31-5. (London: Biological Engineering Society)

13. Cochrane, R. and Sherriff, S.B. (1985). Stimulus-response measurement of skin blood flow by laser Doppler flowmetry - does it provide useful information? In Spence, V.A. and Sheldon, C.D. (eds.) Practical Aspects of Skin Blood Flow. pp 36-41. (London: Biological Engineering Society)

14. Payne, P.A., Faddoul, R.Y. and Jawad, S.M. (1985). A single-channel pulsed Doppler ultrasound instrument for measurement of skin blood flow. In Spence, V.A. and Sheldon, C.D. (eds.) Practical Aspects of Skin Blood Flow. pp 18-22. (London: Biological Engineering Society)

15. Faddoul, R.Y. (1985). A high frequency ultrasound pulsed Doppler system for the measurement of skin blood flow. PhD thesis. University of Manchester (UMIST)

16. Nilsson, G.E., Tenland, T. and Oberg, P.A. (1980). Evaluation of a laser Doppler flowmeter for measurement of tissue blood flow. IEE Trans. Biomed. Eng., **BME-27**, 597-605

Chapter 14

The structure and pathophysiology of skin lymphatics

T J Ryan

Dermatologists have ignored the subject of lymphology in almost every discussion of the biology of the skin and failed to give any emphasis to lymphatics. This is partly because they are difficult to see and early workers concentrated on descriptions of the more visible lymphatics of the viscera. Skin lymphatics are, in fact, rather large vessels with extremely attenuated walls principally lying as two plexuses - one just below the subpapillary venous plexus of the upper dermis, and the other in the deep dermis and the fat. Normally these lymphatic vessels are collapsed and empty. Indeed, a dilated lymphatic is often an indication of malfunction. In order to study the distribution of the lymphatics it is sometimes helpful to obstruct their outflow as may be done in the skin of the pig[1]. Following the making of an island flap in pig skin, the lymphatics are widely dilated and can be seen to be clearly different to the smaller blood vessels since their endothelium is extremely attenuated whereas the endothelium of smaller blood vessels is plump and prominent. Valves are frequent in the lymphatics of the upper and mid-dermis, but there are no valves in small blood vessels except in the deepest parts of the dermis. Dilated lymphatics lie close enough to the surface to be occasionally visible to the naked eye in fair skin and some investigators use fluorescein-labelled dextran to show up the superficial plexus in human skin[2].

THE DEVELOPMENT OF LYMPHATICS

In the embryo, blood vessels develop from primitive mesenchymal cells or angioblasts, and the blood vessels are clearly differentiated from lymphatics by the properties of the vessel wall. The cardiovascular system requires that the developing blood vessel is able to resist blood pressure so as to prevent excessive leakage, and to have a lining which is adapted to platelets, the coagulation cascade and other blood factors. Thus the endothelium of the blood vessels secretes many agents concerned with fibrinolysis and platelet disaggregation. It is an organ which carefully controls its permeability and builds a wall commensurate with the degree of pressure within the vessel. Some leakage of water and macro-molecules, nevertheless, occurs into the interstitium and has to be removed. Pockets of such fluid collect in the tissues and are immediately surrounded by mesenchymal cells which eventually form the lymphatic. Lymphatic endothelium is initially only a lining cell, around boluses of fluid, eventually providing a system which will return protein to the cardiovascular system. It is a system well endowed with valves with no basal lamina or adventitial cells in its wall. Pressure within the lymphatic is very low and the endothelium is lacking any system to effectively deal with coagulation and platelets. It is, nevertheless, a system which can adapt, and in diseased states, it is likely that the lymphatic endothelium finds itself in new environments formed by the leakage of blood into the tissues or the development of a higher pressure within the lymphatic. This is a case of endothelial adaptation so that the lymphatic endothelium is less easily distinguished from blood vessel endothelium.

ELASTIC FIBRE NETWORK

The lymphatic system has to respond to movement in the surrounding tissues. Having virtually no spontaneous pulsation at capillary level, the only way it can clear its contents is by responding to the movement of surrounding tissues. These include vibration, massage and arterial pulsation. Ryan[3] and Mortimer et al.[1] believed that an elastic network was an essential part of the lymphatic system in the skin enabling it to respond to such movements. Since Unna's description in 1896[4] there have been observations on the elastic fibre network surrounding lymphatics in the skin[3] but the full significance of this network has been ignored. Using an orcein stain one can show that the elastic network not only surrounds the initial lymphatics (Figure 14.1a) but is anchored to surrounding tissues such as the collagen and even the epidermis[5] (Figure 14.1b). In vivo techniques such as the injection of colloidal carbon into the skin suggest that the elastic fibre network may also be a pathway by which macromolecules can pass into the lymphatics. This is an observation previously made by Hauck in his studies of mesentery interstitium[6]. The orientation of elastic fibres within the dermis is predominantly vertical in the papillary dermis and horizontal in the reticular dermis. The relationship of this network to the lymphatics has been the subject of a study in the Oxford department[5] which suggests that the dermal lymphatics may be preferentially orientated in the direction of Langer's lines.

STUDIES OF LYMPHATIC FUNCTION

Previous workers studying lymphatic function in the skin have assumed that the lymphatics should be studied in the immobilized tissue. Many workers have been concerned with showing the lymphatic trunks rather than the initial pathways and therefore the injections of any materials they have used to demonstrate lymphatics have been subcutaneous rather than carefully in the neighbourhood of the initial lymphatics. Mortimer et al.[7] in this department have performed a number of controlled studies showing that high

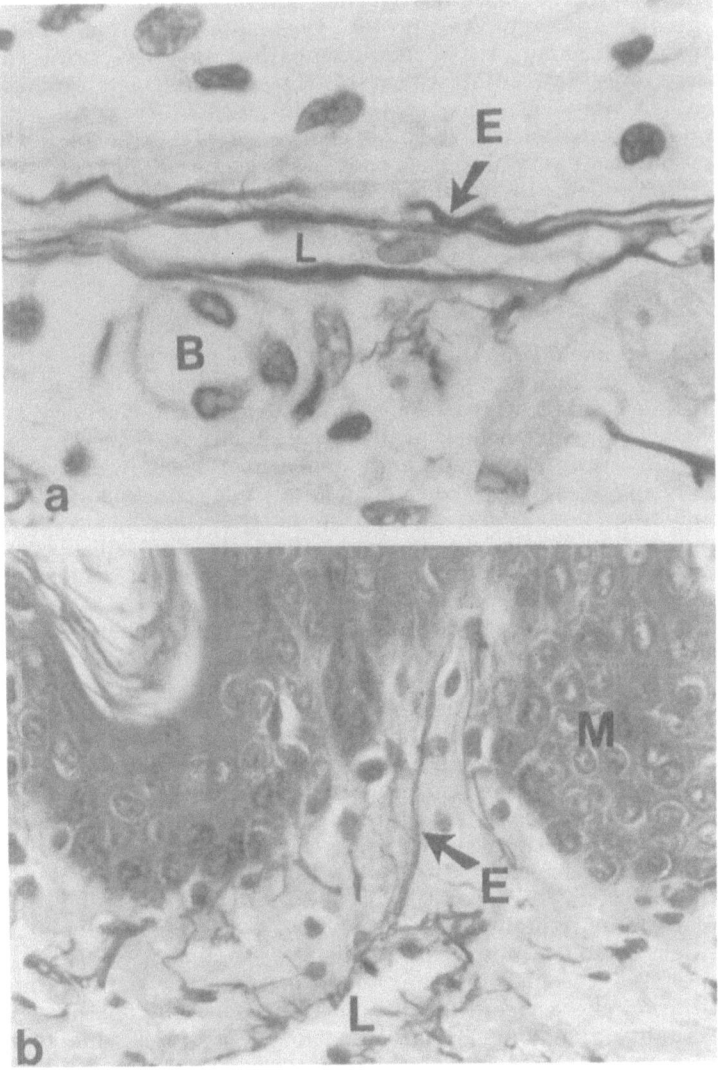

Figure 14.1 (a) An initial lymphatic (L) surrounded by elastic fibres (E). An adjacent blood capillary (B) is devoid of elastic fibres (magnification = X 1500); (b) An initial lymphatic (L) in the upper dermis is surrounded by elastic fibres, some of which are seen passing up towards, and inserting into the dermal-epidermal junction (E). M = epidermis (magnification = X 800). Stain: orcein. (Courtesy of R Jones)

intradermal injection of very small amounts of macromolecules is a prerequisite for accurate estimation of lymphatic function in the skin. They have used technetium colloid and inject only 0.03 ml. Furthermore, they have shown that lymphatics in the immobilized limb function very incompletely and that the proper study of the lymphatic system requires movement. Mortimer and colleagues have used gentle massage to effect lymphatic function and have demonstrated clearly that the lymphatics in the skin function effectively only in the presence of movement. Their studies have included not only clearance of technetium colloid from the skin but the uptake within the lymph node. A feature of lymphatic dysfunction is that while clearance may occur locally by diffusion within the tissues, in lymphoedema pathways to the lymph node are grossly inefficient.

LYMPHOEDEMA

Lymphoedema should be defined as a consequence of a mechanical insufficiency of lymph drainage[8]. The main causes of lymphoedema in the United Kingdom are cancer and surgical interference such as post-mastectomy lymphoedema. A classification therefore can be divided into cancer-related and non-cancer-related. Non-cancer-related lymphoedema may be congenital; it can also be due to infections and toxins and the latter is the commonest reason for lymphoedema in tropical countries, filariasis and silica-containing contamination of the skin being the two principal causes of the worldwide problem.

An important concept is the idea that lymphoedema can result from exhaustion of the lymphatic system, overstressed by an exceedingly vulnerable venous system. Thus, it is probable that every case of venous disease of the lower legs results in some degree from lymphatic malfunction. The consequences of lymphoedema are many and in particular they include the organization of protein within the tissues and eventual fibrosis, but they also result in change in the oncotic pressure in the tissues so that the normal physiology of the interstitium is grossly disturbed. A further important consequence of lymphatic failure is the failure to clear antigenic protein and inflammatory cells from the tissues, particularly recirculating T cell lymphocytes[8]. Not only is the interstitium affected but the epithelial tissues are grossly disturbed as well as the vascular and nervous elements that pass through the interstitium. The concept of lymphostatic haemangiopathy suggests the possibility that arteriosclerosis changes could be due to damage to vessel walls consequent on a failure to clear protein and macromolecules. Currently, it is my belief that many chronic inflammatory disorders of the lower leg, including nodular vasculitis, can be explained by the accumulation of white cells as a consequence of failure of clearance. Moyses et al.[9] have shown that in the standing position white cells pass out of the capillaries of the lower leg. If the lymphatics are unable to respond to an excess of white cells in the tissues then conditions of white cell accumulation are inevitable and are most likely to occur at the dermal subcutaneous border. One characteristic pattern of pathology resulting from this sequence is nodular vasculitis.

CONCLUSION

Lymphatic channels are a vital component of the cutaneous microcirculation. Although largely ignored by skin biologists in the past, it is becoming clear that they can be readily identified and studied from the functional point of view. Data on their involvement in the pathophysiology of inflammatory skin disorders are also emerging.

REFERENCES

1. Mortimer, P.S., Cherry, G.W., Jones, R.L., Barnhill, R.L. and Ryan, T.J. (1983). The importance of elastic fibres in skin lymphatics. Br. J. Dermatol., **108**, 561
2. Jager, K. and Bollinger, A. (1985). Fluorescence microlymphography, technique and morphology. In Bollinger, A., Partsch, H. and Wolfe, J.H.N. (eds.) The Initial Lymphatics. (Stuttgart: George Thieme Verlag)
3. Ryan, T.J. (1978). The lymphatics of the skin. In Jarrett, A. (ed.) The Physiology and Pathophysiology of the Skin. Vol.5, 2nd edn., p. 1755. (London: Academic Press)
4. Unna, P.G. (1896). The Histopathology of the Diseases of the Skin. (Edinburgh: William F Clay)
5. Jones, R.L. (1985). Elastic fibres and the lymphatics: a light microscopical study of their functional association in normal and leprous skin. FIMLS Thesis, Institute of Medical Laboratory Sciences, London
6. Hauck, G. (1982). The connective tissue space in view of lymphology. Experientia, **38**, 1121
7. Mortimer, P.S., Young, C.M.A. and Ryan, T.J. (1985). Characterisation of lymph flow by simultaneous and continuous monitoring of depot clearance and nodal uptake using Tc^{99m} labelled colloid. In Casley-Smith, J.R. and Piller, N.B. (eds.) Progress in Lymphology: Proceedings of the Xth International Congress of Lymphology (Adelaide). p. 132 (South Australia: University of Adelaide)
8. Olszewski, W. (1985). Peripheral Lymph: Formation and Immune Function. (Boca Raton, Florida: CRC Press)
9. Moyses, C., Cederholm-Williams, S.A., Ledingham, J.G.G. and Michel, C.C. (1985). Sequestration of white cells in the feet during sitting. Int. Microcirc: Clin. Exp., **4**, 294

Chapter 15

The physical basis for cutaneous sensation

A Compston

In primitive organisms, the nervous system enables movement within the environment; in turn, this requires information about the boundary between self and the outside world which is provided by sensation. At a higher level of organization, sensation also registers internal environmental changes. Skin and some internal structures are therefore endowed with a rich sensory neural network, which has, as its main function, protection against noxious stimuli. This was recognized by early physiologists such as Rene Descartes[1].

The importance of nocioception can be seen in patients who lack pain sensation, leading to mutilation of the analgesic extremities, seen for example in hereditary sensory neuropathies, or of internal structures, especially joints, occurring in diabetes, syringomyelia or neurosyphilis. But associated with these protective properties of sensation and depending on them for its higher order organization, is discriminative sensation. The consequence of alteration in this form of sensation on function, especially in the arm, is much greater than mere weakness or cutaneous sensory loss and results in an almost useless hand in which the ability to carry out organized movements such as writing, dressing or picking up small objects is lost.

Clinical neurology has devised a method for examining sensation which identifies patterns of sensory loss from which disease is localized and its cause predicted. To this end, clinicians assess sensory modalities regarded as functionally distinct; these include touch, pain, temperature, pressure, vibration, compound sensations such as tickle and itch and discriminative or proprioceptive modalities subserving awareness of position sense, kinaesthesia, shape, texture and two-point threshold. Examination of these sensations is coupled with anatomical knowledge of the different pathways through which individual modalities are conducted within the peripheral nervous system, spinal cord, brainstem, thalamus and parietal cortex. Skin contains receptors subserving awareness of touch (Meissner, Merkel's discs, and nerve terminals around hairs), pain (beaded nerve heads and nerve fibres around blood vessels), pressure (Pacinian), warmth (Rufini) and cold (Krause). Peripheral nerve contains myelinated (A) and non-myelinated (C) fibres; each may be large or small and conduction velocity varies directly with size. A fibres are further classified depending on conduction velocities seen in the compound action potential into alpha, beta, gamma and delta neurons. A delta and C fibres are thought to conduct pain; other peripheral neurons are also modality specific.

Sensory loss is distal and symmetrical in peripheral neuropathy, whereas a localized area lacks sensation in individual nerve injuries. Some anatomical rearrangement of fibres occurs in the dorsal nerve roots, producing the dermatomal patterns of sensory loss; the size of individual modalities depends on the degree of overlap between adjacent roots. But stereotyped patterns of sensory loss are seen most clearly in spinal cord disease; diagnosis is based on the principle that fibres subserving pain, temperature and crude touch enter via the dorsal root entry zone, ascend a few segments, decussate and further ascend in the spinothalamic tract. Fibres subserving discriminative forms of sensation ascend ipsilaterally in the cuneate (sacral, lumbar and thoracic) and gracile (cervical) tracts in the posterior columns to the medulla where they decussate joining the spinothalamic tract to form the medial lemniscus. Facial sensation enters the brainstem via the three trigeminal divisions into a long ipsilateral trigeminal nucleus and thereafter decussates as the quintothalamic tract. Thus, all sensation from one half of the body eventually reaches the opposite thalamus. From there it projects through a compact bundle of fibres in the internal capsule to the parietal cortex.

Using a minimum of equipment and this anatomical knowledge, clinicians can distinguish patterns of sensory loss arising from peripheral nerves (glove and stocking), roots (dermatomes), spinal cord (e.g. Brown-Sequard syndrome), medulla (lateral medullary syndrome), thalamus (hemisensory loss), and cortex where parts are represented depending on their functional requirements depicted by Penfield and Rasmussen as the sensory homunculus[2].

This is the stimulus-specific network of sensation originating with Descartes and later developed by von Frey. But clinicians easily become frustrated by this scheme and in clinical practice frequently have to interpret apparently conflicting sensory signs; vibration sense is often preserved in severe posterior column disease, position sense is retained in patients with severe sensory wandering, and positive cutaneous sensory symptoms such as burning, tightness or painful dysaesthesiae occur in posterior column disease. The concept of a modality-specific chain of connecting neurons subserving sensation also does not easily explain pain referred either from a diseased structure to a distant point on the skin, or to another part of the body, after cutaneous stimulation in an area rendered analgesic by cordotomy. Modality-specific theories also cannot explain the phenomenon of phantom pain. At first the amputee is aware of a tingling phantom which has an appropriate shape and movement. Later, the connecting limb may disappear leaving a suspended extremity which eventually telescopes into the stump. Tingling alters to pain, warmth or heaviness usually disappears but can persist to a disabling degree in a minority of patients. The pain may be referred into the phantom from other cutaneous zones, or normal visceral sensations such as bowel and bladder emptying. The pain is refractory to therapeutic procedures within the central nervous system, but can be relieved temporarily by local injections of saline and anaesthetic, or by sympathectomy. Causalgia is similar in intensity and intractability to phantom pain and usually complicates partial trauma to the median or sciatic nerves; this was first described by Weir Mitchell after the American Civil War[3]. The pain is provoked by sensations in the affected part, which are normally soothing, or unrelated stimuli such as noise and startle; it also can improve after local procedures which affect sensory input, especially sympathectomy.

Damage to dorsal root ganglia by herpes zoster also leads to excruciating pain with many clinical features of causalgia and the same is true of spontaneous pains occurring in trigeminal neuralgia. These syndromes all display marked summation of cutaneous stimuli, increase in the presence of auditory or emotional disturbances, show delays in perception, spread outside the stimulated area and are resistant to surgical control but may be relieved by modification of sensory input. None of these syndromes can be explained by theories of unidirectional modality-specific sensation.

In some normal individuals pain is not perceived because of the circumstances in which it occurs; for example, emotional factors may inhibit awareness of pain during heroic acts, and sporting injuries are commonly ignored during the game. Denial of pain is not uncommon in neurological practice and is usually identified because the parts apparently involved do not conform to recognized patterns of sensory loss based on anatomical principles.

It was against this background that new concepts emerged of the physical basis for sensation. The first to propose an alternative to the unidirectional chain of connected neurons was Henry Head who arranged for James Sherren to cut and resuture his superficial radial and lateral cutaneous nerves in the forearm. The recovery pattern was described by Rivers and Head[4]; adopting Hughlings-Jackson's ideas on hierarchies in the nervous system they proposed that sensations were either deep, protopathic (primitive and crude sensations) or epicritic (discriminatory sensations); the latter were thought to be subserved exclusively by the posterior columns. A recent critic has pointed out that Head's theories led to the conclusions that when a thermal stimulus is applied after cordotomy, the patient would feel nothing but nevertheless, know where it was[5]. If Head did no more than question existing theories, the pendulum swung full circle with Weddell's pattern theory[6] borrowing from Aristotle's idea that pain is the experience of any excessive sensation. Weddell and colleagues concluded that no individual fibre type is concerned with a particular sensory modality; the spatial and temporal discharge patterns of peripheral fibres and their central connections provide the full range of sensory experience. According to this theory, one fibre can transmit information about several sensations. Weddell took as his starting point the finding that von Frey's basic sensations (hot, cold, pain and touch) can each be appreciated in parts of the skin where the putative receptors are not present, especially in the cornea where only one type of nerve ending exists. It has also been concluded that many of the histological entities previously assigned individual functions are merely structures that develop with ageing. But although pattern theory may be correct for visceral sensation, it is perhaps too non-specific to account for the peripheral basis of cutaneous sensation. More recent ideas accept some specificity in function of skin receptors and afferent peripheral nerve fibres.

Cutaneous sensory receptors can be defined morphologically and classified[7] to include rapidly adapting mechanoreceptors responding to an alteration of as little as 1 μm and these include the Pacinian corpuscles (vibration), hair follicles and field receptors. There are slowly adapting cutaneous mechanoreceptors (types 1 and 2), equivalent to Rufini endings; these have myelinated afferent fibre connections. In addition there are non-myelinated mechanoreceptors that do not conduct cutaneous responses. Meissner corpuscles, with their myelinated afferent nerve fibres, and Merkel cells (found only in glabrous skin) are equivalent to the fast and slowly adapting receptors. Thermo-receptors have non-myelinated fibres and are evidently neither Krause nor Rufini structures. Nocioceptors consist of mechanoreceptors which fire in response to pinch or prick and are connected to small myelinated and non-myelinated fibres whereas other nocioceptors are responsive to extremes of temperature.

However, these stimulus-specific properties are not assigned any significance in the gate control pattern theory proposed by Melzack and Wall[8]. They propose that access to central pathways depends on activity in hypothetical T cells, located in Rexed's lamina V of the spinal cord. Input to this cell is 'gated'. In permitting transmission or not of peripheral impulses subserving pain, T cells are inhibited or facilitated first by descending central pathways and secondly through the balance of afferent discharge in large myelinated and small unmyelinated fibres themselves. These influences on the T cell are coordinated through the substantia gelatinosa. Excess activity in small fibres opens the gate and causes pain whereas large fibre firing inhibits T cells and closes the gate. If activity is balanced, the gate is ajar. Criticisms of the theory are based on clinical and experimental considerations[5]. Specifically, clinicopathological predictions of the theory are not met in practice. Whilst in post-herpetic neuralgia there is usually the large fibre loss predicted by the gate theory and thermoanalgesia occurs in the small fibre demyelination seen in amyloid neuropathy, most large fibre neuropathies are painless and some conditions in which there is selective small fibre loss are painful. The improvement in intractable pain predicted by the gate theory following percutaneous nerve stimulation is observed in clinical practice, even though large fibre stimulation does not selectively reduce pain.

In response to criticisms, Wall[9] modified the theory and conceded that impulses concerning injury reach the spinal cord or trigeminal nucleus via A delta and C fibres and receiving cells are additionally facilitated or inhibited by other peripheral fibres or descending central control systems. Pre- and post-synaptic gating is thus achieved by integration of primary signals, other afferent sensory impulses and descending controls.

The most significant recent addition to understanding sensory theory has been recognition that activity in the peripheral and central nervous system is influenced by neurotransmitters[10]. Their role and interactions are not yet fully established but there is evidence that the dorsal horn area of spinal cord, connecting with C fibres, is rich in substance P and this may be the major pain neurotransmitter. Gate control could involve inhibition of substance P by adjacent neurons requiring encephalins as transmitters and in turn, these connections may be facilitated by descending serotoninergic neurons. The otherwise unexplained influence of the sympathetic nervous system on pain pathways may also have as its basis sensitivity of damaged peripheral neurons, or structures within the dorsal horn region of spinal cord, to local concentrations of catecholamines and other sensory neuropeptides.

The physical basis for sensation is complicated and not yet fully understood, but the existing information is consistent with a general neurological principle which has best been illustrated in the controversy surrounding cerebral localization; lesions can be localized, but function cannot.

REFERENCES

1. Descartes, R. (1662). De homine figuris et latinitate donatus a Florentio Schuylo. (Lugduni Batavorums. F. Moyarduns and P. Leffen)
2. Penfield, W.O. and Rasmussen, T. (1950). The Cerebral Cortex of Man. p. 44. (New York: Macmillan)
3. Mitchell, S.W. (1872). Injuries of Nerves and Their Consequences. pp. 292-6. (Philadelphia: Lippincott and Co.)
4. Rivers, W.H.R. and Head, H. (1908). A human experiment in nerve division. Brain, 31, 323-450
5. Nathan, P.W. (1976). The gate-control theory of pain. Brain, 99, 123-58
6. Weddell, G., Palmer, F. and Paillie, W. (1955). Nerve endings in mammalian skin. Biol. Rev., 30, 159-95
7. Iggo, A. (1971). Cutaneous and subcutaneous sense organs. Br. Med. Bull., 33(2), 97-102
8. Melzak, R. and Wall, P.D. (1965). Pain mechanisms: a new theory. Science, 150, 971
9. Wall, P.D. (1978). The gate control theory of pain mechanisms. Brain, 101, 1-18
10. Iverson, L.L. (1982). Substance P. Br. Med. Bull., 38(3), 277-82

Section V

MECHANICAL PROPERTIES

Chapter 16

The physical properties and function of nails

A Y Finlay

Nails are not only an evolutionary hangover from our ancestors' jungle-life. We continue to make use of our nails as weapons, as tools, for body care and as social ornaments. The functions of nails, however, depend on their physical properties which in turn are directly dependent on their gross anatomical structure, their cellular structure and hence on their biochemical components.

A wide variety of physical properties of nails can be measured; it is useful to identify those properties which are of any practical relevance, to allow relevant objective measurements to be made of changes in nails in disease states. As a weapon for pinching, scratching or tearing, longitudinal strength and sharpness are necessary, but nails must not be brittle. When used as a tool, such as forceps, screwdriver or scraper, lateral strength, hardness and lack of upward bending are additional advantages. Renewability and durability against friction forces are also essential.

Flexibility, hardness and the ability to act as a buttress are all of importance in the body care functions of scratching, grooming, removing splinters or picking teeth. Finally because of the physical properties of smoothness, shininess and non-flaking, nails are decorated and used socially to try to increase attractiveness. Examples of these functions are illustrated in Figures 16.1-8.

Although toenails are of little functional value, fingernails have a variety of functions even in the industrial age; we **do** use them (see Table 16.1). They are only useful, however, because of their physical properties which may be altered by disease such as psoriasis or by the action of drugs[1]. To gain an objective measure of these physical properties, a variety of adaptations of standard methods of measurement have been applied to nails, and totally new devices have been built to measure specific physical properties. Most of these techniques have been applied in vitro; the relevance of this testing has been challenged[2], but testing in vivo poses major practical difficulties. There are also problems in describing exactly what properties of nail are of relevance to measure and in defining some of the terms used: for example there is considerable overlap between 'flexibility', 'hardness' and 'strength'.

This review focuses solely on the physical properties of nail plate, and ignores ingenious methods for measuring properties of even very closely attached tissue[3]. Dawber and Baran[4] give a wider review of the structure of nail, and an excellent further short review of nail physical properties.

Table 16.1 Practical functions of nails

Functions	Example	Physical properties needed
Weapon		
Pinch	Aggressive fighting	⎧ Longitudinal strength
Scratch		⎨ Sharpness
Tear		⎩ Lack of brittleness
Tool		
Cutlery	As a knife	⎧ Lateral strength
Forceps (Figure 16.1)	For fine gripping	⎪ Hardness
Scraper (Figure 16.2)	To scrape off surface of coated games	⎨ Lack of upward bending
Screwdriver (Figure 16.3)	Unscrewing locks	⎪ Durability against friction forces
Edge detector	To amplify feel of uneven surface	⎪ Renewability
Picker (Figure 16.4)	To aid picking up small objects	
Plucker (Figure 16.5)	Playing the guitar	
Body care		
Scratcher	Can add to damage of inflamed skin	⎧ 'Buttress'
Squeezer	Helps 'spot squeezing'	⎨ Low flexibility
Toothpick (Figure 16.6)	Method for removing matter stuck between teeth	⎩ Hardness
Grooming (Figure 16.7)	Instant comb	
Splinter remover (Figure 16.8)	First aid tool	
Nosepick	Nails essential	
Social/aesthetic		
Decoration site	Mainly females	⎧ Non-flaking
Intimate behaviour	To amplify a caress	⎨ Smooth

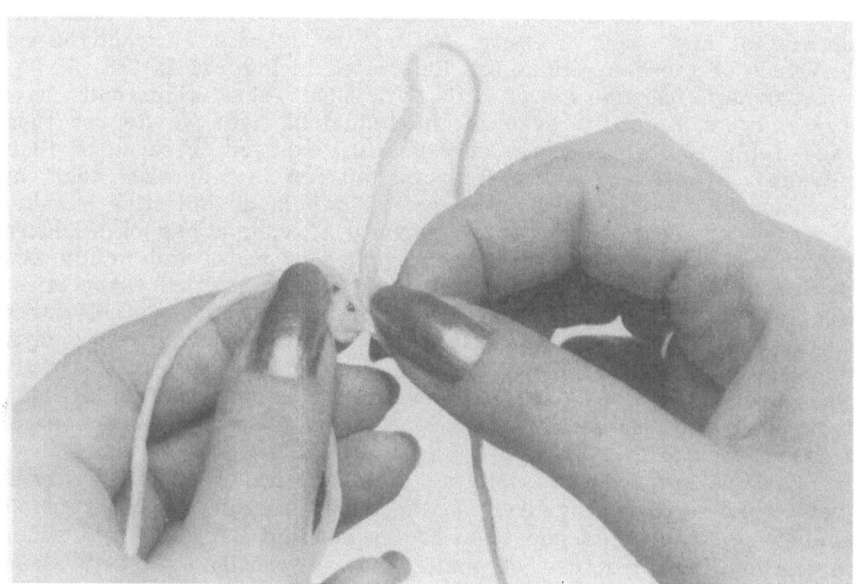

Figure 16.1 Forceps

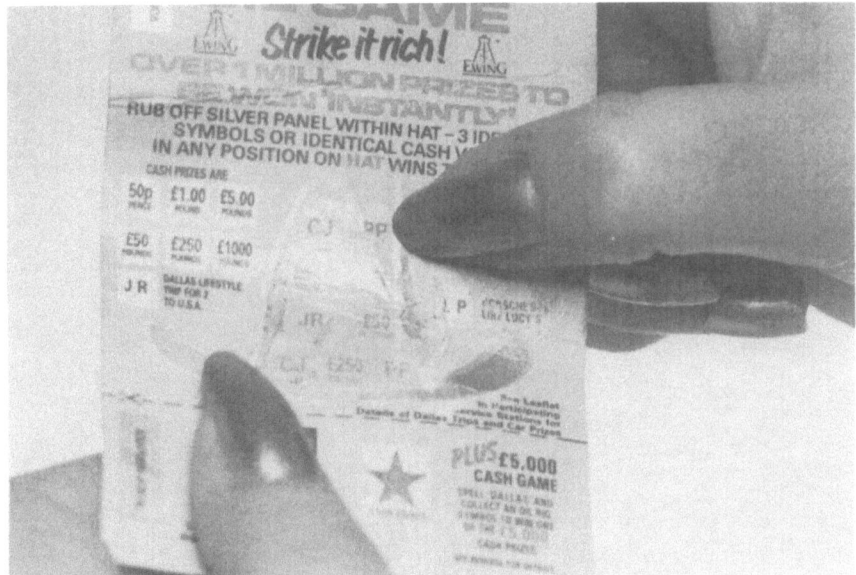

Figure 16.2 Scraper

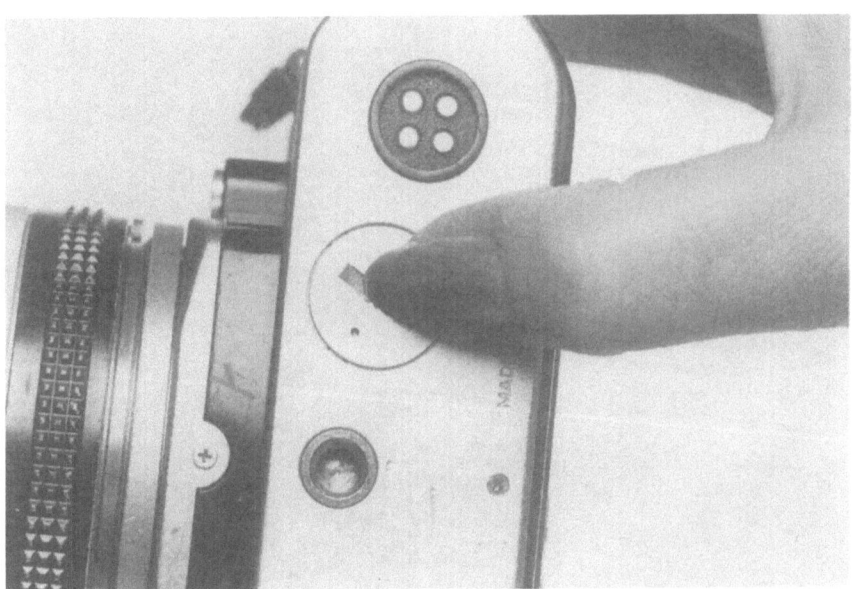

Figure 16.3 Screwdriver

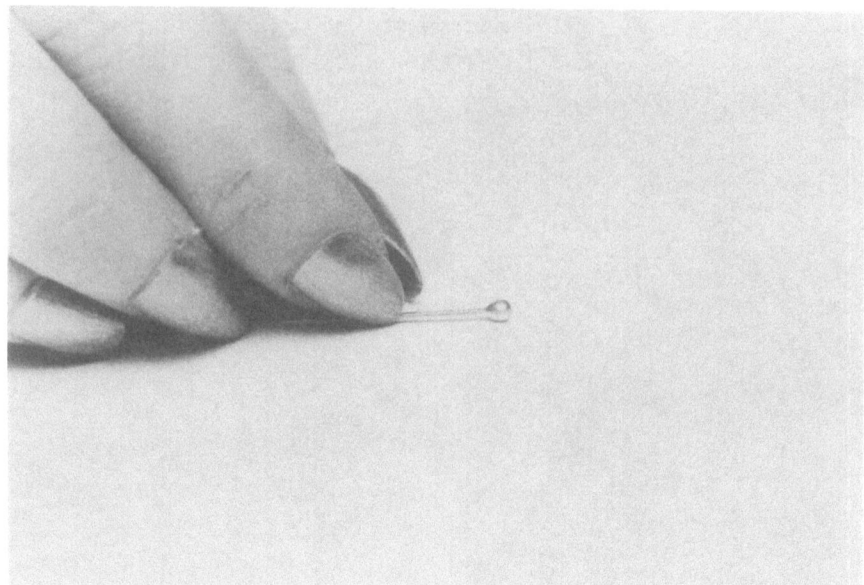

Figure 16.4 Picker

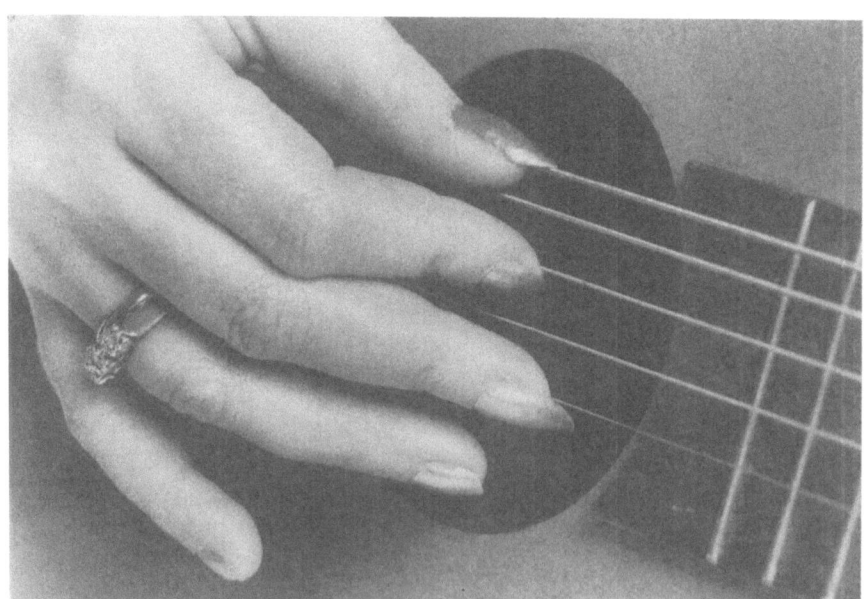

Figure 16.5 Plucker

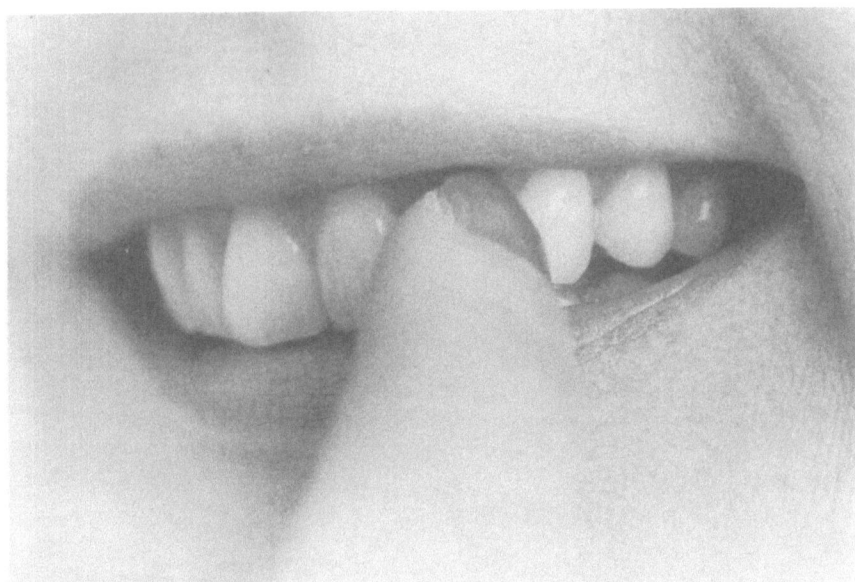

Figure 16.6 Toothpick

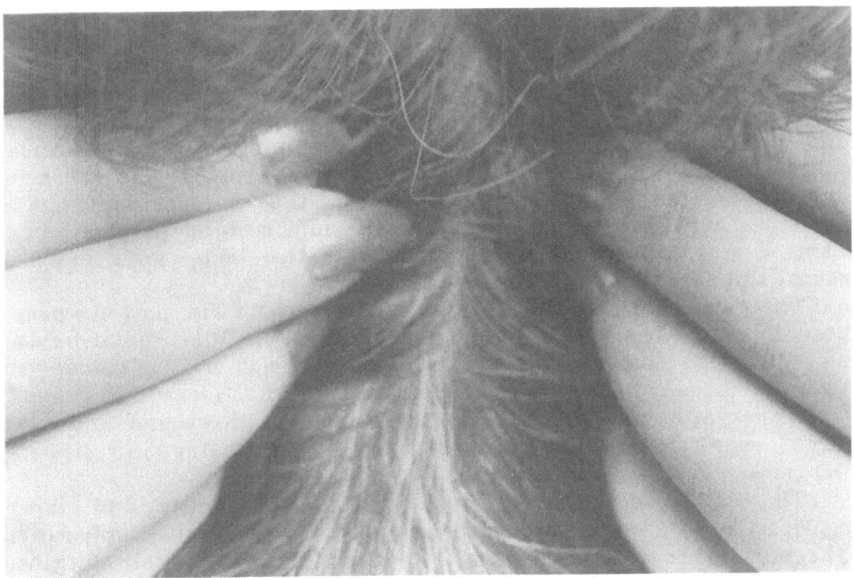

Figure 16.7 Grooming

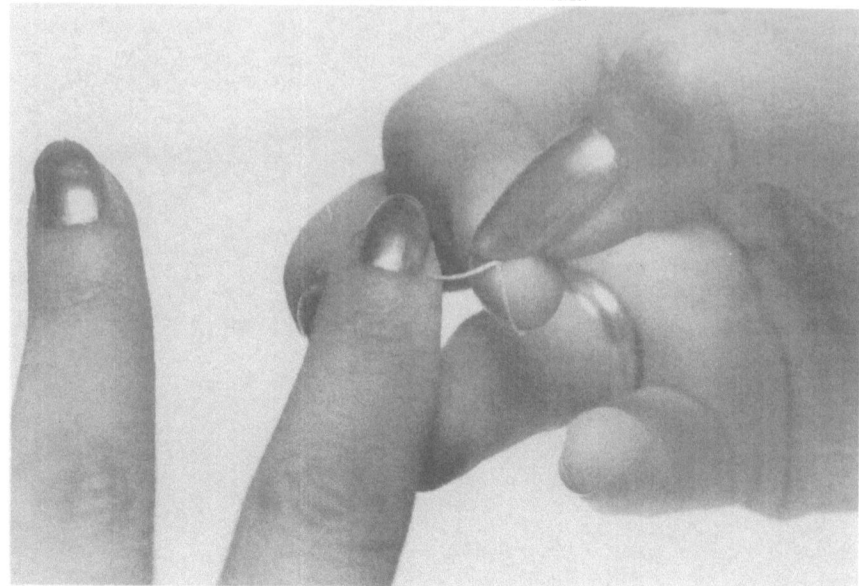

Figure 16.8 Splinter remover

NAIL ANATOMY

The nail plate is usually curved in one plane and often in two. This shape confers on a nail additional strength to withstand external injury. Further strength is gained by the integration of the drier and hence harder 'outer shell', the dorsal nail plate, and the more hydrated softer ventral nail plate[5]. In this respect nail has a structure analogous to the 'ever-sharp' knife made of parallel layers of hard and soft steel, the thicker soft steel being worn away to reveal thinner, sharp, hard steel.

The thumbnail and index fingernail are the nails most commonly used for the variety of functions given in Table 16.1. As increased nail thickness confers greater strength on a nail it is advantageous that the thumbnail and index fingernails are the thickest fingernails both proximally and distally, as measured by ultrasound and by a direct micrometer method (Finlay, Moseley and Duggan, Br. J. Dermatol., in press).

The ability of nails to grow and be constantly and slowly replaced is an obvious but important property of the nail apparatus. The wide range of functional uses of nails carries the risk of trauma and damage and so replacement rather than permanent loss is an advantage. Meyer and Grundmann[6] have suggested that the nail while growing shifts over the nail bed as if on railway tracks, and have observed complimentary grooves and ridges on the ventral surface of avulsed nail plate and on the nail bed.

Although the functional requirements of the nail alter little with age, there clearly are age-related changes in nail structure.

Corneocytes of the dorsal nail plate increase in size with age[7] and fingernails tend to become thicker as age increases (Finlay, Moseley and Duggan).

NAIL CONTENT

Although not strictly a physical property of nail, the structural components and elemental contents clearly form the physical basis for the way in which nail plate behaves. Protein content is of prime importance to the strength of nail but it is the detection of minute quantities of other substances that has exercised the minds of forensic scientists, paediatricians, diabetologists, haematologists and beauty specialists. Trace metal content in normal nail has been measured by Alexiou et al.[8] and Bauer[9]. ABO (H) blood group substances are detectable in nails[10] and changes in chloride content and glycosylation have been measured in cystic fibrosis and diabetes[11,12]. Detective novel enthusiasts will have guessed that the arsenic content of nails has been measured[13] but as nail does not have the resilience of hair to long-term burial degradation, nail arsenic content is unlikely to be of relevance in postmortem exhumations.

Nail is formed from differentiated keratinocytes produced by that specialized area of epidermis, the nail matrix. These dead keratinocytes contain a matrix with tightly packed keratin filaments with a diameter of 7-10 nm[14]. There seems to be no difference in the structure and orientation of the cornified cells from the harder dorsal nail plate and the softer ventral nail plate.

Both nail and hair contain a mixture of proteins in a filament-matrix structure which is stabilized by disulphide bonds. The constituent proteins of human hair and nail are essentially the same although their relative proportions are different, with nail containing less high sulphur proteins. Genetic variation has been noted in the low sulphur and high sulphur protein fractions[15]. In addition, small differences have been noted in the low sulphur proteins of hair and nail in the same individual[16].

Nail matrix stays in situ for many months after its formation, up to ten times longer than epidermis. Time-related changes may therefore partly explain differences in protein content[17], as there may be degradation of low molecular proteins within nail.

X-ray diffraction studies show that the keratin fibril orientation is in the flat plane of the nail surface, orientated mainly at right angles to the direction of growth. This gives lateral reinforcement, preventing longitudinal cleavage of the nail[18]. In contrast, in hair the protein filaments are parallel to the growth axis[19]. Nail and hair, in contrast to stratum corneum, contain a non-helical component very rich in cysteine[20].

HARDNESS

Although the concept of hardness is immediately understandable, there are several different measuring techniques and each technique defines hardness differently. Classically, hardness assessment depended on the ability of a material to withstand scratching from a range of objects of different hardness, but now hardness tests usually depend on assessment of depth of indentation caused by a defined shape and force.

The water content of nail is the single most important factor influencing nail hardness, as the reader will be aware from personal experience of bathtime nail cutting. During water immersion, nail takes up to 22% of its original weight within 2 hours[21] and its flexibility increases in parallel. The establishing of standard conditions of humidity and water content are crucial, therefore, to gaining meaningful measurements of nail hardness. Generally tests of hardness have been carried out on the dorsal surface of nails. It should be borne in mind, however, that nail is probably not uniform in its water content and so ventral nail is likely to be less hard than dorsal nail.

Michaelson and Huntsman[22] used a Knoop (pyramidal-diamond) indentor to demonstrate that nail hardness may be increased by gelatin intake. Robson[23], in an 'airnail' link-up study between the Philippines and Michigan, also used a Knoop indentor to show that in children nail hardness may be related to nutritional status. Newman and Young[24], however, clearly illustrated the range of practical and environmental problems inherent in measuring nail indentation hardness, and concluded that fingernail hardness is in the range of many commercial plastics (about 20-40 Knoop). One of the major difficulties in repeatedly measuring nail hardness is the necessity for securing nail firmly against a non-compressible base; the shape of nail clippings makes securing difficult and the mattress effect of the underlying dermis makes this testing virtually impossible in vivo. Further variation results from the indentor causing unrecoverable deformation because of the rheological properties of nail keratin[24].

A different approach was used by Ramrakhiani[25] who measured spherical ball indentation of nail by an optical method. Full recovery of local indentation of nail took up to 1 hour.

RIGIDITY, FLEXIBILITY AND STRENGTH

Realizing that hardness tests were not ideal, Young et al.[26] carried out basic flexural tests on nail, producing load-deflection curves for nail specimens compressed centrally over a span. The range of maximum stress varies from 4.2 to 8.2 x 10^6 Pa, similar to strength values for horse hair, wool and human hair. The measurement of Young's modulus (no relation) of nail provides a standard measure to compare the 'springiness' of nail to other materials in a standard fashion. Baden[19] used two different techniques to measure Young's modulus; a standard measurement of deflection with varying load ($3-5 \times 10^{-13}$ N m^{-1}) and measurement of velocity of sound in nail from which the modulus can be calculated.

Nail exhibits viscous flow at loading and so Forslind et al.[27,28] also felt that 'hardness' is not an appropriate label for the property of withstanding breaking and buckling but 'rigidity' or 'stiffness' would be more exact. They measured the effective elastic modulus of nail under a variety of environmental conditions and again stressed the importance of water content on nail physical properties.

Finlay et al.[21] described an instrument which repeatedly flexed nail sections until they fractured. This study demonstrated the direct relationship of flexibility to nail water content, and the importance of phospholipid content in maintaining nail flexibility.

In a creative study Maloney et al.[29] miniaturized a number of different standard devices for testing nail physical properties. They recorded the following ranges of physical properties; flexural strength, $3.5-11.7 \times 10^7$ N m^{-2}; tensile strength, $2.8-11.7 \times 10^7$ N m^{-2}; tearing resistance, $4.8-12.0 \times 10^3$ kg m^{-1}; and impact absorption (rebound ratio) 0.4-0.7.

BARRIER FUNCTION

An ability to understand the barrier function of nail is now of direct practical relevance in the design of topical drugs to treat nail disease. In 1946 Burch and Winsor[30] used a simple gravimetric method to measure water diffusion through postmortem nail specimens and skin from various body sites, and were the first to demonstrate the surprising finding that diffusion rates through nail were similar to the most rapid palmar and plantar sites. Spruit[31] measured in vivo nail water vapour loss by passing dry nitrogen over nail and measuring the water carried away by the gas, a method previously used for measuring transepidermal water loss. There was a constant inverse relationship between the rate of water vapour loss (2-3 mg cm^{-2} h^{-1}) from nail to its thickness, suggesting that there is no difference in permeability of the dorsal and ventral layers of nail.

More recently Walters et al.[32] have used a diffusion cell to provide detailed information about nail permeability coefficients for water, methanol and ethanol in vitro. They used this method to investigate nail diffusion by measuring diffusion of a variety of n-alkanols with a range of different diffusion and oil-to-water distribution coefficients. Nail becomes less permeable to n-alkanols as their hydrophobicity is increased, and so very polar compounds might more easily pass through nail plate[33].

There are major differences between the permeability characteristics of nail and epidermis, probably due to differences in the relative amounts of lipid and protein; nail contains less than 1% lipid[20]. The barrier behaviour of nail plate is similar to that of a hydrogel of high ionic strength[33]. In stratum corneum the lower permeability of dissociated compounds may be due to an ability of ions to partition into the lipid phase. In nails, however, the low lipid content results in both dissociated and undissociated compounds such as miconazole penetrating nail at equivalent rates[34]. The most important aspect of enhancing drug nail penetration is therefore to improve the solubility of the drug in the vehicle. This may be done by decreasing pH which in nail, though not in stratum corneum, would not adversely affect penetration.

Direct testing of the effects of vehicle on the permeation of drugs[34] points the way to an important theoretical basis for the formulation of drugs and bases with the best characteristics to pass through nail plate. These studies can be complemented with direct measures of penetration of topically applied drug using an in vitro radio-labelling technique. This method has demonstrated the theoretical advantage of using tincture rather than ointment as a vehicle for antifungal agents[35].

RADIATION TRANSMISSION

It is obvious that normal nails can transmit light. There are, however, good practical reasons for being able to measure how well nails do transmit visible light, ultra violet radiation or X-rays. Gammeltoft and Wulf[36], noting that X-rays and Grenz rays have been widely used in the treatment of psoriatic nails, measured in vitro the ability of normal and fungally infected nails to transmit these radiations. There is an inverse correlation between log thickness and transmission of 12 kV Grenz rays: the dose needed therefore to effectively penetrate very thick diseased nails would risk damage of surrounding skin and so this treatment should be reserved for nails of less than 0.9 mm thickness. 29 kV X-rays, however, have better properties of penetration.

Visible light plays a part in the pathogenesis of photo-onycholytic reactions, and the rational use of PUVA to psoriatic nails depends on an understanding of the ability of nail to transmit UVA. Relatively little UVA reaches the nailbed and only radiation > 330 nm is transmitted[37]. About 2.5 times the normal therapeutic dose for skin would be needed for the same effect on the underlying surface of the nail plate.

HEAT CONDUCTIVITY

A curious attempt to use a physical property of nail to estimate accidentally received doses of ionizing radiation was unsuccessful[38]. In theory radiation should induce thermally stimulated currents in fingernail, but unfortunately these changes were so small that they were masked by the ability of nail to rapidly 'leak' the current induced.

CONCLUSION

Human nails are functionally important and have a range of physical properties which allow these functions. Many of these properties can be reproducibly measured, although testing in vivo poses many more problems than in vitro. The ability to measure physical properties in vivo will potentially allow objective measurements of nail in health and disease, and may also be used to assess the effects of different therapeutic measures.

REFERENCES

1. Lindskov, R. (1982). Soft nails after treatment with aromatic retinoids. Arch. Dermatol., **118**, 535-6
2. Dawber, R.P.R. and Finlay, A.Y. (1985). Physical properties of hair and nails: workshop report. Bioeng. Skin, **1**, 57
3. Mahler, F., Muheim, M.H., Intaglietta, M., Bollinger, A. and Anliker, M. (1979). Blood pressure fluctuations in human nailfold capillaries. Am. Phys. Soc., **236**(6) H888-93
4. Dawber, R.P.R. and Baran, R. (1984). Investigations and some physicochemical properties of nails. In Baran, R. and Dawber, R.P.R. (eds.) Disease of the Nails and their Management. Chap. 3, pp 98-102. (Oxford: Blackwell Scientific Publications)
5. Forslind, B. and Thyresson, N. (1975). On the structure of the normal nail. A scanning electron microscope study. Arch. Derm. Forsch., **251**, 199-204
6. Meyer, J.Ch. and Grundmann, H.P. (1984). Scanning electron microscopic investigation of the healthy nail and its surrounding tissue. J. Cut. Path., **11**, 74-9
7. Germann, H., Barran, W. and Plewig, G. (1980). Morphology of corneocytes from human nail plates. J. Invest. Dermatol., **74**, 115-118
8. Alexiou, D., Koutselinis, A., Manolidis, C., Boukis, D., Papadatos, J. and Papadatos, C. (1980). The content of trace elements (Cu,Zn,Fe,Mg) in fingernails of children. Dermatologica, **160**, 380-2
9. Bauer, F. (1983). Investigations of trace metal content of normal and diseased nails. Aust. J. Dermatol., **24**, 127-9
10. Garg, R.K. (1983). Determination of ABO (H) bloodgroup substances from finger/toe nails. Am. J. Forens. Med. Path., **4**, 143-4
11. Chapman, A.L. et al. (1985). X-ray microanalysis of chloride in nails from cystic fibrosis and control patients. Eur. J. Resp. Dis., **66**, 218-23
12. Bakan, E. et al. (1985). Glycosylation of nail in diabetics; possible marker of long-term hypercalcaemia. Clin. Chim. Acta, **147**, 1-5
13. Pounds, C.A. (1979). Arsenic in fingernails. J. Forens. Sci. Soc., **3**, 165-73
14. Caputo, R., Gasparini, G. and Contini, D. (1982). A freeze-fracture study of the human nail plate. Arch. Dermatol. Res., **272**, 117-25
15. Marshall, R.C. (1980). Genetic variation in the proteins of human nail. J. Invest. Dermatol., **75**, 264-9
16. Marshall, R.C. (1983). Characterization of the proteins of human hair and nail by electrophoresis. J. Invest. Dermatol., **80**, 519-24
17. Shono, S. and Toda, K. (1983). The structure proteins of the human nail. In Seiji, M. and Bernstein, I.A. (eds.) Normal and Abnormal Epidermal Differentiation, Current Problems in Dermatology. pp 317-26. (Basel: Karger)
18. Forslind, B., Lindstrom, B. and Philipson, B. (1971). Quantitative microradiography of normal human nail. Acta Dermatovener. (Stockh.). **51**, 89-92
19. Baden, H.P. (1970). The physical properties of nail. J. Invest. Dermatol., **55**, 116-22
20. Baden, H.P., Goldsmith, L.A. and Fleming, B. (1973). A comparative study of the physicochemical properties of human keratinized tissues. Biochem. Biophys. Acta, **322**, 269-78
21. Finlay, A.Y., Frost, P., Keith, A.D. and Snipes, W. (1980). An assessment of factors influencing flexibility of human fingernails. Br. J. Dermatol., **103**, 357-65
22. Michaelson, J.B. and Huntsman, D.J. (1963). New aspects of the effects of gelatin on fingernails. J. Soc. Cosmet. Chem., **14**, 443
23. Robson, J.R.K. (1974). Hardness of finger nails in well-nourished and malnourished populations. Br. J. Nutr., **32**, 389-94

24. Newman, S.B. and Young, R.W. (1967). Indentation hardness of the fingernail. J. Invest. Dermatol., **49**, 103-5
25. Ramrakhiani, M. (1978). Indentation and hardness studies of human nails. Ind. J. Biochem. Biophys., **15**, 341-3
26. Young, R.W., Newman, S.B. and Capott, R.J. (1965). Strength of fingernails. J. Invest. Dermatol., **44**, 358-60
27. Forslind, B. (1970). Biophysical studies of the normal nail. Acta Dermatovener. (Stockh.), **50**, 161-8
28. Forslind, B., Nordstrom, G., Toijer, D. and Eriksson, K. (1980). The rigidity of human fingernails: a biophysical investigation on influencing physical parameters. Acta Dermatovener. (Stockh.), **60**, 217-22
29. Maloney, M.J., Paquette, E.G. and Shansky, A. (1977). The physical properties of fingernails. 1. Apparatus for physical measurements. J. Soc. Cosmet. Chem., **28**, 415-25
30. Burch, G.E. and Winsor, T. (1946). Diffusion of water through dead plantar, palmar and torsal human skin and through toe nails. Arch. Derm. Syph., **53**, 39-41
31. Spruit, D. (1971). Measurement of water vapor loss through human nail in vivo. J. Invest. Dermatol., **56**, 359-61
32. Walters, K.A., Flynn, G.L. and Marvel, J.R. (1981). Physicochemical characterization of the human nail. I. Pressure sealed apparatus for measuring nail plate permeabilities. J. Invest. Dermatol., **76**, 76-9
33. Walters, K.A., Flynn, G.L. and Marvel, J.R. (1983). Physicochemical characterization of the human nail: permeation pattern for water and the homologous alcohols and differences with respect to the stratum corneum. J. Pharm. Pharmacol., **35**, 28-33
34. Walters, K.A., Flynn, G.L. and Marvel, J.R. (1985). Penetration of the human nail plate: the effects of vehicle pH on the permeation of miconazole. J. Pharm. Pharmacol., **37**, 498-9
35. Stuttgen, G. and Bauer, E. (1982). Bioavailability, skin and nail penetration of topically applied antimycotics. Mykosen, **25**, 74-80
36. Gammeltoft, M. and Wulf, H.C. (1980). Transmission of 12 kV Grenz rays and 29 kV X-rays through normal and diseased nails. Acta Dermatovener. (Stockh.), **60**, 431-2
37. Parker, S.G. and Diffey, B.L. (1983). The transmission of optical radiation through human nails. Br. J. Dermatol., **108**, 11-16
38. Grey, L.J. and Bowlt, C. (1978). An attempt to use thermally stimulated currents in human nail to estimate dose in cases of accidental exposure to ionising radiation. Phys. Med. Biol., **23**, 759-60

Chapter 17

Mechanical properties of stratum corneum: influence of water and lipids

J-L Lévêque and L Rasseneur

INTRODUCTION

The stratum corneum (SC) is a thin membrane made up of an agglomerate of long, flat cells in a lipid-rich amorphous material known as 'intercellular cement'. This membrane consists of keratin (about 60%), lipids (about 15%), amorphous proteins (about 15%) and various low-molecular weight substances (about 10%). SC can, therefore, be considered to be a composite membrane, i.e. membrane made up of elements with widely differing properties.

The main function of SC is to provide a limiting barrier across which exchanges can occur between the biologic-medium and the surrounding environment. In vivo, the SC must be able to carry out this vital physiological function despite the distortion and constraint to which it is constantly subjected and in all possible climatic conditions.

It is only because of its remarkable viscoelastic properties, which we will discuss below, that it is able to perform its task effectively.

THE INFLUENCE OF HYDRATION

Blank was the first, in 1952[1], to demonstrate to what extent water could influence the elastic properties of SC. In a dry state, the SC is brittle; when hydrated, it becomes plastic and highly extensible. More precisely, it has been shown that the elastic modulus varies by a coefficient of the order of 100 over the range of 40-100% relative humidity[2] (see Figure 17.1). It should be noted that this finding is in agreement with the data published by Van Duzee[3]. This figure of 100 is markedly greater than that found for hair (about 2.8)[4]. The principal difference between the behaviour of these two types of structure with regard to water is apparent above 70% relative humidity. The capacity of hair to take up water is limited to about 30%, whereas the SC is able to absorb several times its own weight of water (see Figure 17.2).

The types of bonding which exist between water and SC have been discussed in several studies and the findings are summarized in Table 17.1. The findings all indicate that above a water content of approximately 36-40%, the water is present in a freer form, i.e. in a form involving less interaction with the SC structure.

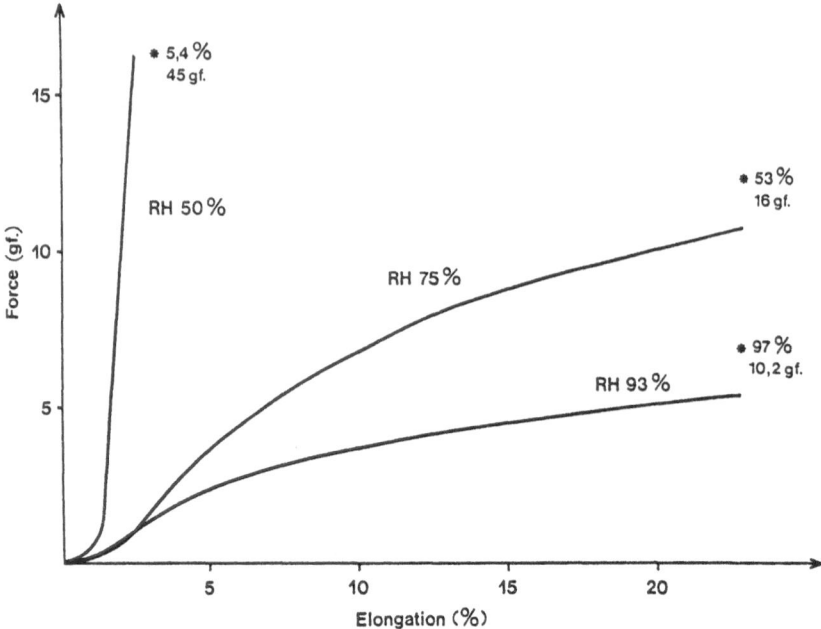

Figure 17.1 Force-elongation diagram of human stratum corneum samples according to the conditioning relative humidity; T_A = 30°C (the asterisk represents the ultimate strain and the force at break)

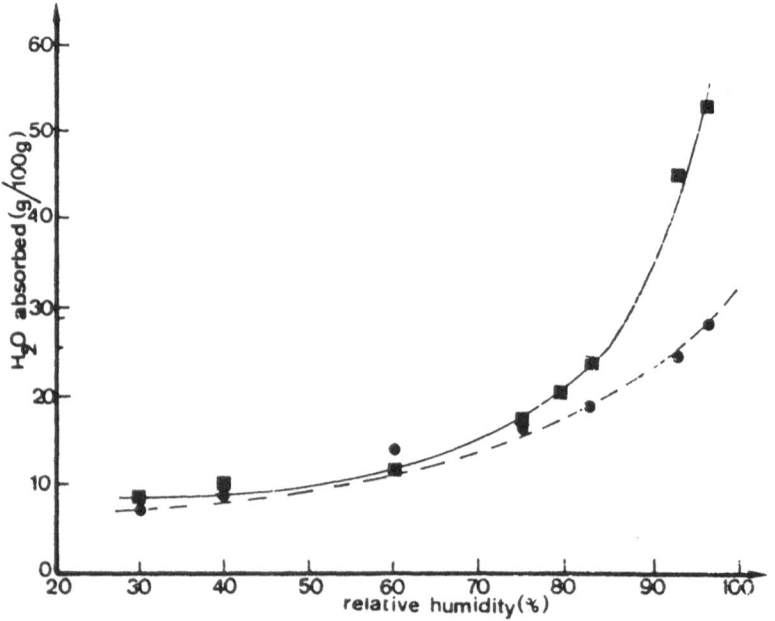

Figure 17.2 Sorption isotherms for stratum corneum (square) and human hair (circle)

Table 17.1 Summary of results concerning the relative amounts of bound and unbound water according to references 14-18

Reference	Methods	Strongly bound water	Bound water	Free water
18	Gravimetric	5-10%	10-500%	> 500%
16	Differential calorimetry		0-34%	> 34%
17	Gravimetric (mathematical analysis)		0-47%	> 47% (intracellular)
15	IR,NMR	10-20%	15-36%	> 36%
14	Gravimetric (mathematical analysis) NMR,X-ray	5-8%	5-36%	> 36%

IR = infra-red; NMR = nuclear magnetic resonance

If a graph is plotted with the water content on the X-axis and the elastic modulus, the electric resistivity or the absorption of the SC at 300 nm on the Y-axis, it is found that these parameters fall rapidly at a content of about 30-40%, which corresponds to the level at which the water is said to be in the 'free' state. In this state, it has less influence on the structure of the SC, and this explains the shallower slope of all these curves in this region[5-7]. In general, water appears to affect the elastic properties of keratin and to act as a plasticizing agent, in the chemical sense of an agent which reduces the interactions between the chains, either by the formation of a hydrogen bond with the peptide group or by shielding the charges between the ionic groups (glutamic acid/lysine, for example).

THE INFLUENCE OF LIPIDS

Figure 17.3 shows the sorption isotherm obtained for delipidized samples. The fact that this curve lies just above the curve obtained with normal SC indicates that the lipids may mask some of the hydrophilic sites of keratin.

Determinations of the elasticity and water content for normal and delipidized samples also show clearly that the lipids have a plasticizing effect on the SC (see Table 17.2).

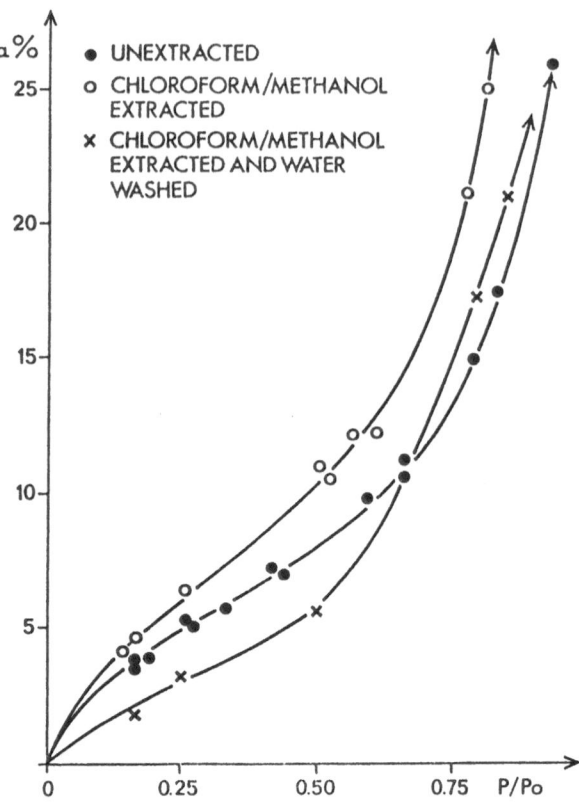

Figure 17.3 Sorption isotherm for stratum corneum; P/Po represents the partial pressure of water vapour

Table 17.2 Correspondence between the Young's modulus (E_d) and the water content of stratum corneum samples measured at 58% and 73% of relative humidity

	58%			73%		
	Unextracted	Extracted	Extracted + water washed	Unextracted	Extracted	Extracted water was
Water content (%)	11.1	12.2	8.3	17.2	20.8	17.2
E_d (10^8 N m^{-2})	5.49 ± 0.23	7.91 ± 0.3	9.77 ± 0.55	2.53 ± 0.1	2.54 ± 0.2	5.62 ± 0
% variation	-	44 ± 4	78 ± 4	-	0 ± 9	122 ± 1

This is an important finding, since the accepted 'dogma' from the time of Blank's findings in the 1950s has been that only water is able to plasticize the SC. In fact, if one looks carefully at the work of Blank and the more recent work of Middleton[8], it can be seen that these authors did, in fact, detect the effect of lipids on the elasticity of the SC, but they did not comment on this finding, probably because the effect of the lipids is weaker than that of water.

If we accept the hypothesis advanced by Elias[9] according to which virtually all the epidermal lipids are contained in the intercellular spaces of the SC, then this implies that they play an important part in controlling the viscoelastic properties of the SC.

INFLUENCE OF HYDROSOLUBLE MATERIALS

When samples of delipidized SC are rinsed in water, about 10-15% (w/w) of soluble substances can be extracted. These substances consisting, amongst others, of free amino acids (see Table 17.3) have been termed 'natural moisturizing factors' (NMF) by Jacobi[10].

Table 17.3 Relative composition of the 'natural moisturizing factors'

Free amino acids	40%
Pyroglutamic acid	12%
Urea	7%
Sodium	5%
Calcium	1.5%
Potassium	4%
Magnesium	1.5%
Phosphates	0.5%
Chlorides	6%
Lactates	12%
Undetermined fractions	8.5%

They have a crucial effect on the hydration of SC (see Figure 17.3) since in the zone of moderate humidity, the delipidized samples of SC which have undergone water extraction have a water content only half that of control specimens.

In addition, the equilibrium kinetics of this process are extremely slow: 24 hours after placing the samples in the controlled humidity and temperature zone, equilibrium has yet to be reached. Thus, not only does the presence of NMF affect the water content, but it also promotes thermodynamic equilibrium between the SC and the environment. In view of the factors discussed in the previous paragraph, it is possible that some of the constituents of NMF are located in the intercellular spaces, as has been suggested by some authors[11].

INFLUENCE OF VARIOUS TREATMENTS

Table 17.4 summarizes the effects of the various treatments which were applied to static and dynamic models of SC. It is difficult to comment on the effects of treatment with thioglycollic acid in terms of specific structural features, because the entire structure as a whole appears to be affected. Treatment with salicylic acid, however, has been investigated under the electron microscope, and found to affect only the intercellular cements and produce an increase in the elastic modulus. This implies that treatment of this type could be used to extract the hydrosoluble substances contained in the intercellular cement[12].

Table 17.4 Influence of different treatments on the static (E_s) and dynamic (E_d) elastic moduli of stratum corneum samples[12] (mean ± SE)

	$\dfrac{\Delta E_s}{E_s}$ (%)	$\dfrac{\Delta E_d}{E_d}$ (%)
Thioglycolic acid 8% aqueous solution pH8 4 hours, water rinsed	-89 ± 43	-30 ± 10
Salicylic acid 10% propylene glycol solution 15 hours, ppg rinsed, water rinsed	156 ± 49	70 ± 11
Sodium lauryl sulphate aqueous solution 8% 10 nm water rinsed	-	21 ± 4
Glycerol 3% aqueous solution (5 mg cm^{-2})	-24 ± 11	-34 ± 5
PcNa 3% aqueous solution (5 mg cm^{-2})	-9 ± 13	-26 ± 4

Comparison of the results obtained when the samples were treated with glycerol and with PcNa (the sodium salt of pyroglutamic acid) shows that, under these experimental conditions, the most strongly hydrophilic substance does not produce the greatest effect. The plasticization of SC by water, or by some other substance, can be produced only if the plasticizing agent enters the structure. It is known that glycerol is a molecule which penetrates well into the skin, unlike PcNa which, being a salt, penetrates less well (A Rougier, personal communication). It should be recalled that, according to some authors, glycerol may have a plasticizing effect on intercellular lipids.

CONCLUSIONS

There have been several studies on the viscoelastic properties of the stratum corneum in the past 30 years. During this time, it has been above all the major effects of water molecules on these properties which have been described and discussed. More recent studies have shown that some other molecules, such as urea, for instance, are also able to plasticize the structure of the SC[3]. Other authors demonstrate the indirect role of lipids in the protection of hydrosoluble agents and their direct role in modulating elasticity[5].

This final point is important, because this could explain how it is that the SC is a relatively extensible membrane, even though the cells of which it is made up are relatively resistant to deformation[13].

It should be pointed out that the exact mechanisms by which the factors known as NMF actually act remains unclear in many respects. Thus, 30 years after the important study of Blank, only limited progress has been made in our understanding of the internal mechanisms which confer on the SC its highly remarkable properties, and many important questions still remain unanswered.

REFERENCES

1. Blank, I.M. (1952). Factors which influence the water content of the stratum corneum. J. Invest. Dermatol., **18**, 433-40
2. Park, A.C. and Baddiel, C.B. (1972). Rheology of stratum corneum. A molecular interpretation of the stress-strain curve. J. Soc. Cosmet. Chem., **23**, 3-12
3. Van Duzee, B.F. (1978). The influence of water content, chemical treatment and temperature on the rheological properties of stratum corneum. J. Invest. Dermatol., **71**, 140
4. Fraser, R.D.B. (1972). In Kugelmass, I.N. (ed.) Keratins. (Springfield, USA: C.C.Thomas)
5. Leveque, J.L., Escoubez, M. and Rassneur, L. (1987). Water-keratin interaction in human stratum corneum. (In press)
6. Campbell, S.D., Kraning, K.K., Schibli, E.G. and Momii, T.S. (1977). Hydration characteristics and electrical resistivity of stratum corneum using a non invasive four point electrode method. J. Invest. Dermatol., **69**, 290-5
7. Deffond, D., Leveque, J.L., Scot, J. and Saint-Leger, D. (1985). A photoacoustic investigation of the influence of some constituents of the stratum corneum on ultraviolet absorption. Photodermatology, **2**, 279-87
8. Middleton, J.D. (1968). The mechanism of water binding in stratum corneum. Br. J. Dermatol., **80**, 437-50
9. Elias, P.M. (1981). Epidermal lipids, membrane and keratinisation. Int. J. Dermatol., **20**, 1-19
10. Jacobi, O.K. (1959). About the mechanism of moisture regulation in the horny layer of skin. Proc. Scient. Sect. Toilet Goods Assoc., **31**, 22-9
11. Park, A.C. and Baddiel, C.B. (1972). The effect of saturated salt solutions on the elastic properties of stratum corneum. J. Soc. Cosmet. Chem., **23**, 471-9
12. Rassneur, L., De Rigal, J. and Leveque, J.L. (1982). Influence des différents constituants de la couche cornée sur son module d'élascticité. Int. J. Cosmet. Sci., **4**, 247-60
13. Leveque, J.L., Poelman, M.C. and De Rigal, J. and Kligman, A.M. (1988). Are corneocytes elastic? Dermatologica, 176, 2, (to be published)
14. Hey, M.J., Taylor, D.J. and Derbyshire, W. (1978). Water sorption by human callus. Biochem. Biophy. Acta, **540**, 518-33
15. Hansen, J.R. and Yellin, W. (1972). NMR and infra-red spectroscopic studies of stratum corneum hydration. In Jellinek. Water Structure and the Water-Polymer Interface. (London: Plenum)
16. Walkley, K. (1972). Bound water in stratum corneum measured by differential scanning calorimetry. J. Invest. Dermatol., **59**, 225-31
17. Anderson, R.L., Cassidy, J.M., Hansen, J.R. and Yellin, W. (1972). Hydration of stratum corneum. Biopolymers, **12**, 2789-802
18. Scheuplein, R.J. and Morgan, L.J. (1967). Bound water in keratin membranes measured by a microbalance technique. Nature (London), **214**, 456-8

Chapter 18

The architectural organization and function of the macromolecules in the dermis

Ch M Lapière, B V Nusgens, G E Pierard

+The physiological roles of the dermis are multiple and are mainly dependent on the organization of polymers of macromolecules. Polymeric collagen provides resistance, the unfolding of the collagen bundles attached to the network of elastic fibres allows some mobility, and the viscous hydrated proteo- and glycosaminoglycans give structure to the extracellular fluid where diffusion takes place.

All connective tissues including the two sections of the dermis and the hypodermis are made of similar macromolecules. The main difference between them resides in the architectural organization of these building blocks that will determine the functional properties. Tendons that transmit unidirectional forces are composed of thick bundles of parallel collagen fibres; the transparent cornea is made of a 'plywood' organization of very regular thin fibrils. The dermis, which can be moved in all directions, is supported by a multi-directional undulating network of bundles of fibres with a different architecture in its various sections.

The structure-function relationships can be reproduced at the cellular and molecular level in vitro. Heritable disorders affecting defined macromolecules provide models that support the involvement of different steps in the processing of the macromolecular polymers involved.

MORPHOLOGY OF THE DERMIS AND MECHANICAL PROPERTIES

The connective tissue of the skin can be divided into three parts displaying different architectural organizations of their constituent polymers, namely the adventitial dermis, the reticular dermis and the hypodermis[1]. They are interconnected, establishing a continuous network running from the basement membrane to the underlying fascia and periosteum[2,3].

The papillary dermis supports the undulation of the basement membrane (Figure 18.1). It is formed of thin bundles of collagen fibres almost linear and perpendicular to the basement membrane (Figure 18.2). This network is interwoven with that of elastic fibres including the elaunin and oxytalan fibres, the latter being connected with the lamina densa[4]. The most superficial collagen fibres are tangential to the basement membrane (Figure 18.3) and glide into loops of anchoring fibrils[5].

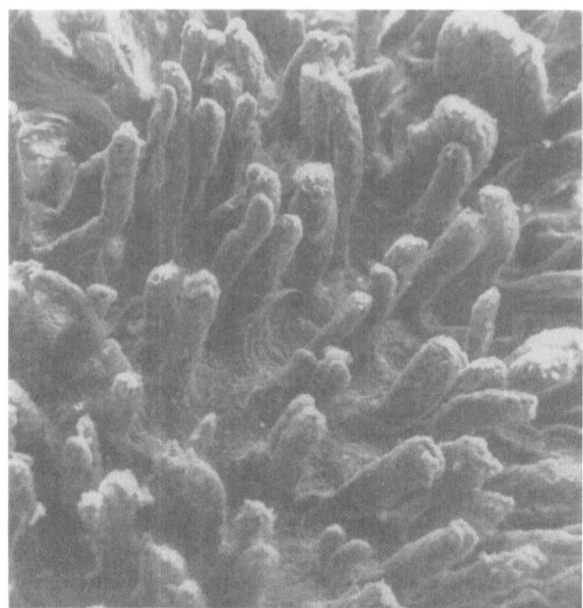

Figure 18.1 Papillated dermo-epidermal junction after separation of the epidermis by sodium bromide

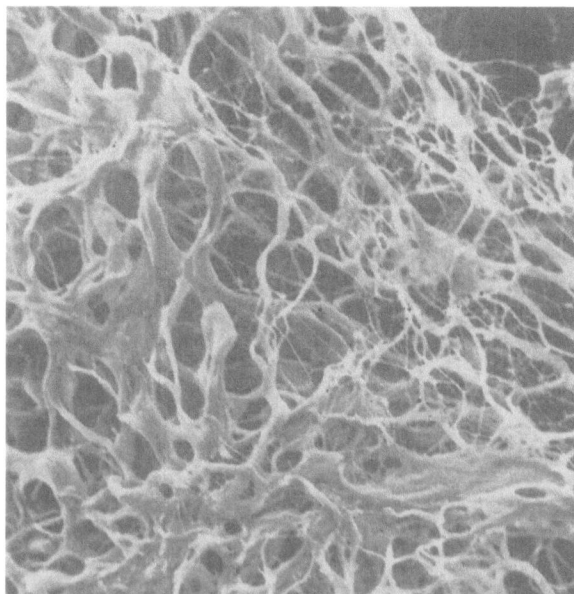

Figure 18.2 Open networks of fibres in the papillary dermis. Thin collagen bundles and elastic fibres are intermingled. Their predominant orientation is parallel to the axis of the dermal papilla

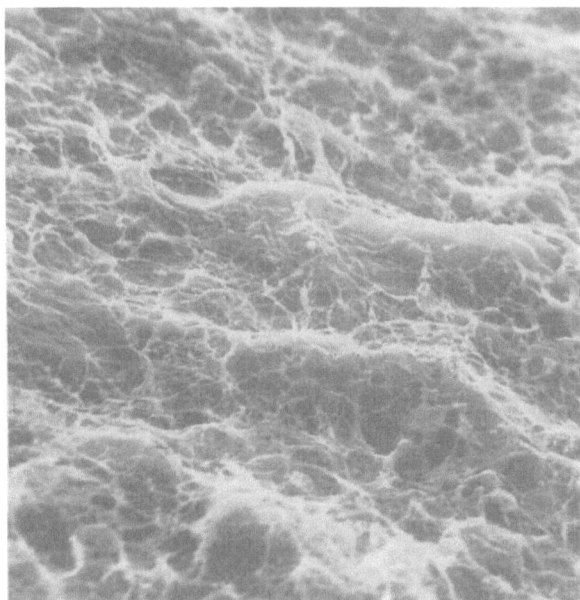

Figure 18.3 Underface of the dermo-epidermal basement membrane. A thin network of fibres is running underneath the membrane

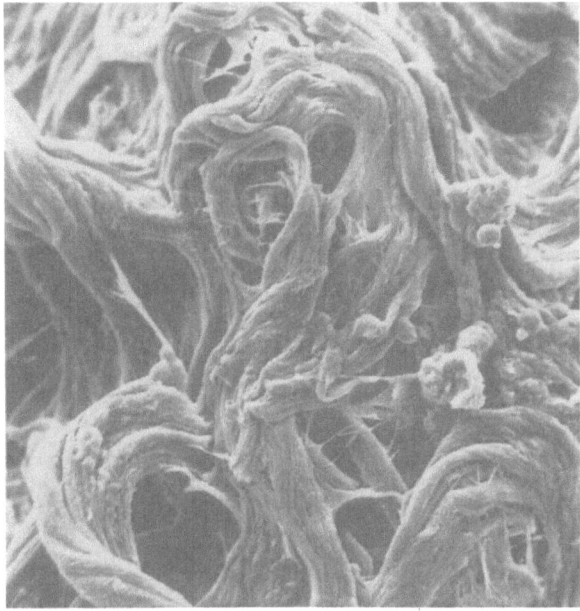

Figure 18.4 Dense network of collagen bundles in the mid-reticular dermis with some elastic fibres in the concavities of the bundles

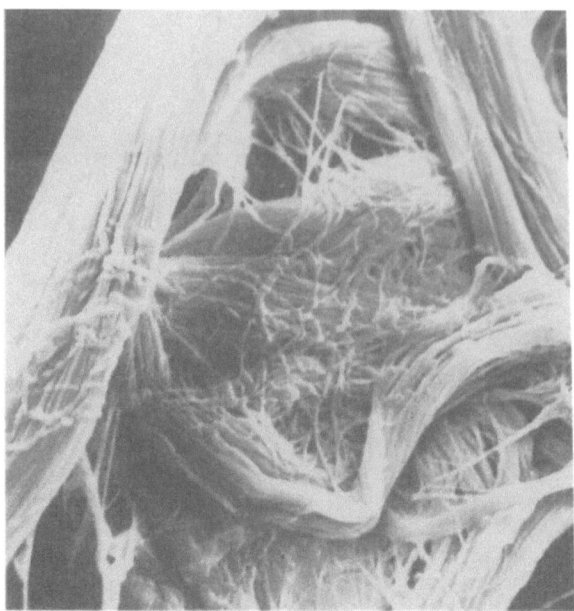

Figure 18.5 Anchorage of collagen bundles one upon another in the reticular dermis

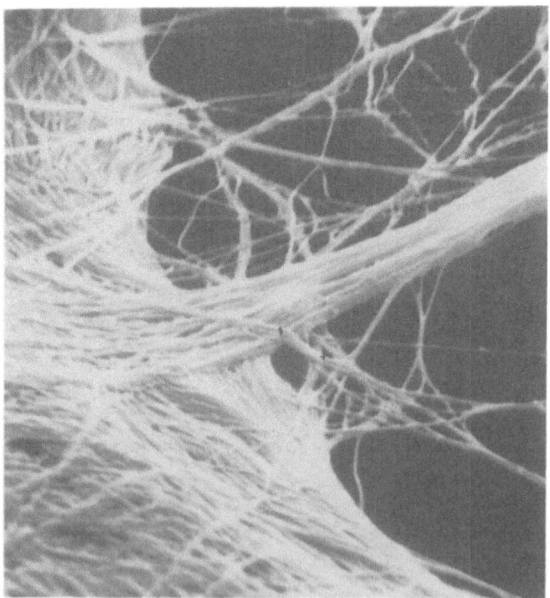

Figure 18.6 Sheet of collagen fibres forming the septa of the subcutaneous fat

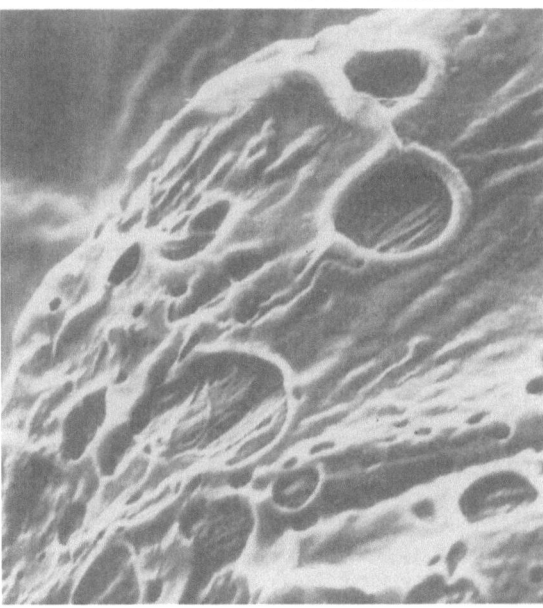

Figure 18.7   Sheath of proteoglycans covering collagen bundles in the reticular dermis

The reticular dermis (Figure 18.4) is made of thick undulating bundles of collagen fibres oriented almost in parallel to the plane of the epidermis. The bundles are connected to each other at multiple points by the interlacing of their fibres (Figures 18.4 and 5). The waviness is supported by the network of elastic fibres. Smaller bundles also ensure the vertical cohesion.

The hypodermis is composed of sheets of interlacing collagen fibres surrounding the adipocytes (Figure 18.6) extending from the deeper part of the reticular dermis to the underlying structures of the skin.

The fibrillar networks of the different sections are barely identifiable by scanning electron microscopy without digestion of the macromolecules of the extrafibrillar space (Figure 18.7). Fibres and cells are indeed surrounded by a highly hydrated and viscous solution of proteo- and glycosaminoglycans.

The rheological properties of the different sections of the dermis depend mainly on the architectural organization of the polymeric macromolecules and on their density[6]. In response to force, all the structures of the dermis will be progressively recruited. The thin straight bundles of collagen in the papillary dermis embedded in the ground substance hold up the dermal papillae. The waviness of the large bundles in the reticular dermis will give little resistance to unfolding since the elastic fibres can be extensively stretched by small force[7-9]. Their Young's modulus is approximately 2×10^5 Pa. The vertical sheets in the hypodermis are extended somewhat by the fat and allow some lateral and vertical movement upon pulling.

The extensibility of polymeric collagen, fibres or bundles of fibres is small[10]. Their Young's modulus reaches 10^9 Pa. The first sign of mechanical failure will occur at a force exceeding the resistance of the small bundles joining the larger bundles. The ultimate force before rupture of the skin will be many orders of magnitude larger and breaking will occur by disruption of the connection between the fibres in the bundles and finally the slipping of the molecules upon one another in the fibres.

It can be safely accepted that the rheological properties of the dermis in the physiological range of forces depend mainly on the organization of the bundles of collagen fibres, the changes in entropy of the elastic network and the viscosity of the extrafibrillar space.

THE MECHANICAL FUNCTION AND THE MACROMOLECULAR COMPOSITION

At least six different types of collagen are present in skin[11]. They participate in their polymeric form in different functions and can be classified as fibrillar for types I and III, microfibrillar for type V, VI and VII and cell membrane-associated for type IV.

The network of elastic fibres is composed of a core of microfibrils supporting elastin, a hydrophobic protein present in large proportion in the elastic fibres, in low amount in the elaunin fibres and alone in the oxytalan fibres[12].

The fibrocyte of the dermis also synthesizes and secretes fibronectin, a large macromolecule composed of multiple functional domains displaying affinity for the cell membrane, heparin and heparan sulphate, collagen, fibrin, hyaluronic acid, DNA and itself[13]. Proteoglycans such as proteodermatan sulphate, chondroitin sulphate as well as hyaluronic acid are released by the fibrocyte to fill the extrafibrillar space. Proteodermatan sulphate, which binds to the collagen fibrils[14], might ensure physical links between the fibrils in the bundles. In vitro, two other types of proteoheparan sulphate have been shown to be produced also by fibroblasts, one probably included in the cell membrane and the other secreted and deposited in the pericellular space[15].

The thickest bundles of fibrils are formed by polymers of collagen type I. They are most abundant in resistant connective tissues such as skin, bone and tendon. The ultimate resistance of skin to rupture is related to this type of collagen. Indeed in dermatosparaxis, a heritable disorder in the calf, polymerization of collagen type I is disturbed by the lack of excision of a precursor peptide and skin is most fragile[16]. Collagen type III, also 'embryonic' or 'vascular', is associated with and probably surrounds the thicker bundles of polymeric collagen type I. The proportion of collagen type III is higher in skin during fetal development and diminishes to reach a constant value from the newborn to the eldest age[17]. During fetal development the architectural organization of the collagen bundles shifts from a pattern found in fish skin (parallel fibres in one plane with a change in orientation in the adjacent planes) to a pattern found in adult mammals[18]. A similar orthogonal 'plywood' organization also occurs in the cornea which contains, besides type I, some collagen types III and V but a large proportion of collagen type VI[19]. Measured by chemical methods in human and bovine skin, the papillary dermis synthesizes a slightly higher proportion of collagen III than the reticular dermis[20]. In both, however, approximately 70% of the collagen is type I. The microfibrillar types of collagen account for less than 5%. By immunofluorescence the labelling of collagen type III is more intense in the papillary dermis, probably because the bundles of fibres are much smaller than elsewhere[21]. The involvement of collagen type III in the development of skin is supported by observations in the Ehlers-Danlos type IV, a genetic disorder characterized by the lack of production of this collagen. In this disease, the skin is very thin and the blood vessels are fragile[22].

Collagen type IV is always associated with basement membrane, a thin and highly folded structure in skin that is most effective in association with its glycoproteins (laminin, entactin, and proteo-heparan sulphate) for the anchoring of epithelial and endothelial cells. The involvement of basement membrane in the overall mechanical properties of skin is probably minor. Collagen type VII makes up the filaments anchoring the basement membrane to the papillary dermis[23]. Their reduction is a cause of mechanical blistering. Collagen type VI seems to participate in the junction between the cells and the fibres and between the fibrils within the bundles. Collagen type V forms very thin polymers interspersed in the space outside of the large bundles[24].

The physical properties of elastin and its high content of polyfunctional cross-links allow it to form a network with a high biological elasticity. It is polymerized within a network of micro-fibrils[25]. In cutis laxa the elastic fibres are ruptured, the skin is lax and the recoil after stretching is slow. The network of bundles of collagen fibres is also extensively modified[6,26]. In the Ehlers-Danlos type I the skin is thin but can be greatly extended. After releasing the tension the skin rapidly regains its initial position. In dermis in this disorder the bundles of collagen fibrils are thin and disorganized while the network of elastic fibres is unchanged and apparently increased relative to the polymeric collagen[27]. The high recoil activity is performed by a well-developed network of elastic fibres acting upon a disrupted framework of bundles of collagen fibrils. These observations support the hypothesis that the network of elastic fibres interwoven with the bundles of collagen fibres allows the latter to keep and regain their wavy pattern ensuring therefore the biological elasticity of the tissue.

The hydration of the dermis is related to the filling of the extrafibrillar space by highly hydrated proteo- and glycosamino-glycans. The space occupied by these very large macromolecules (probably several million daltons) is much smaller in the tissue than in a free solution and their negative charges promote their unfolding[28]. This physical property explains the turgor of the dermis.

Several proteoglycans and glycoproteins secreted by the fibrocytes display other physical functions that are most important at the tissue level. The interaction between proteoglycans and collagen fibrils might be involved in the control of calcium deposition[29]. Fibronectin might be responsible for cell-fibres inter-action[13]. Some cell membrane-associated proteoheperan sulphate might mediate a similar function[30]. These cell-support interactions are most significant in transmitting to the cells mechanical stimuli regulating their biosynthetic activity[31].

MECHANISMS OF FORMATION OF COLLAGEN FIBRES AND THE ORGANIZATION OF BUNDLES

The information required for the polymerization and stabilization of the polymers is contained within well-defined specific domains of the various macromolecules. The mechanism responsible for the association of fibres in bundles and the spatial organization of the network is still hypothetical although some potential controls have been observed in vitro.

Size of the bundles

The post-translational enzyme-mediated modifications of the secreted collagen precursor could condition the size of the fibrils and their capacity to form bundles. Polymerization in vitro of N-terminal extended procollagen results in thin bundles as opposed to the thick bundles obtained by polymerizing fully processed collagen type I[32]. If the C-terminal precursor peptide is excised first the fibrils will be thin while they will be thick if the N-terminal extension is removed first[33].

In vitro the size of the bundles will depend on many physical parameters influencing polymerization such as concentration of the macromolecules, temperature, ionic environment and the presence of other macromolecules such as the glycosaminoglycans[34].

The proportion of the different types of collagen forming the polymers will affect their association. The higher the proportion of type III the thinner will be the bundles as illustrated in Figure 18.8. The influence of this parameter occurs within the range of concentration known to exist in the dermis, up to 30% of collagen type III[35]. It can be said that high mechanical resistance, as in tendon, is associated with the presence of thick bundles of mostly collagen type I while mobility, as in blood vessels, is associated with thin bundles of collagen types I and III. These observations also apply to pathological conditions as in scar formation.

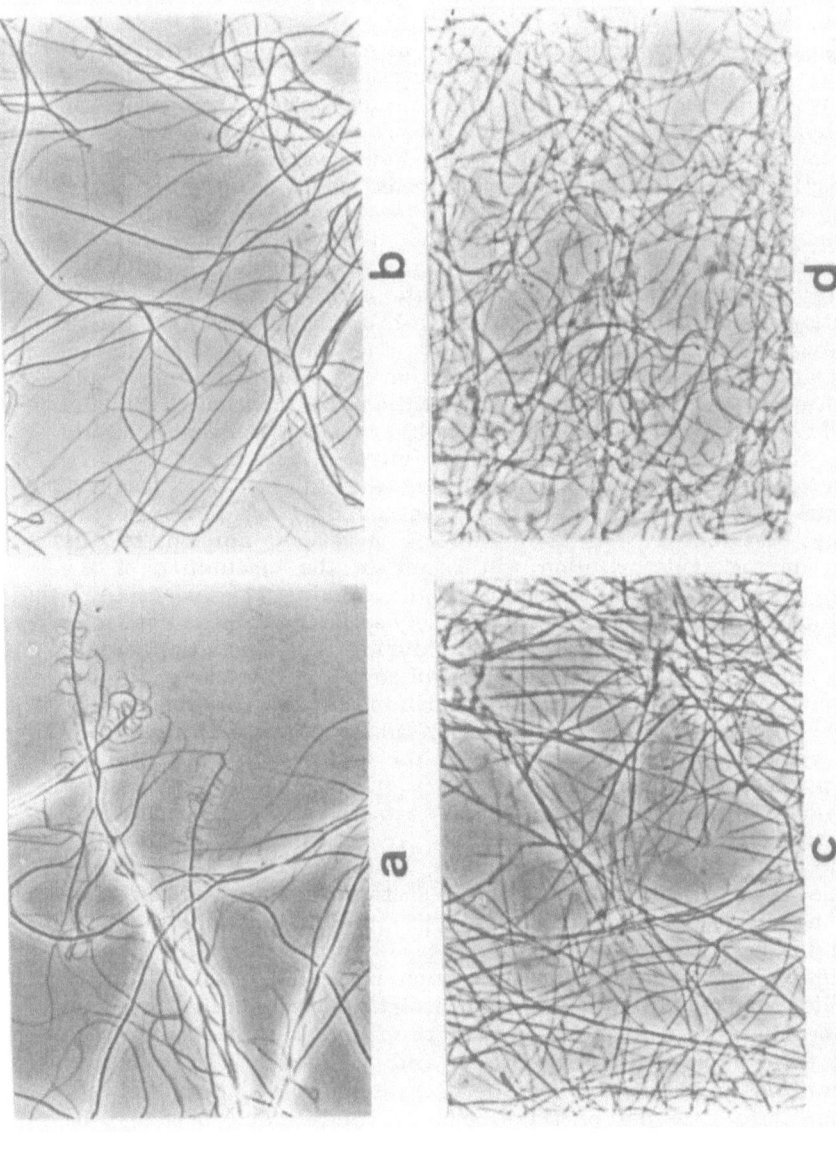

Figure 18.8 Polymerization in vitro of collagen type I and type III in different proportions. The collagens have been extracted from fetal calf skin, fractionated and purified as described in ref.33 and kept in solution at 4°C, 0.15 mg/ml in 0.15 mol/l NaCl at pH 7.4. Polymer formation was obtained by raising to 37°C their films of (a) pure collagen type I, (b) a mixture (V/V) of 97% type I and 3% type III, (c) 90% type I and 10% type III, and (d) 70% type I and 30% type III. For a similar concentration of collagen and a complete polymerization the network of fibres becomes denser when type III increases while the thickness of the bundles is progressively reduced. Phase contrast microscopy x 1200

Direction of the bundles

Obviously, the bundles of polymers in all connective tissues are organized in such a way as to resist specific types of mechanical stresses.

It is known that cells display an asymmetrical distribution of organelles related to a polarized secretion as in the cells of secreting endocrine or exocrine glands. The same also occurs in mesenchymal cells[36]. It has been shown that polymer formation starts in the immediate vicinity of the cell membrane, even within recesses[37]. By such a mechanism cells could contribute to a spatially defined polymerization.

The mechanical forces transmitted from the framework of polymers to the extrafibrillar space might create channels of lower viscosity in the hyaluronic acid gel into which soluble precursors would flow. Collagen is an asymmetrical macromolecule that forms polymers by lateral aggregation and the process depends on concentration. The sieving effect of the glycosaminoglycans could contribute to orientation of polymerization by concentration and alignment of the molecules. A somewhat similar mechanism could explain the following observation in vitro. Polymerization of a solution of native monomeric collagen by warming at 37°C leads to the formation of a gel in which the bundles of polymers are randomly distributed. A unidirectional movement applied to the solution during polymerization will result in the orientation of the polymers parallel with the direction of the shaking (Figure 18.9)[38]. A solution that is shaken before polymerization does not form aligned polymers. It indicates that during polymerization intermediary forms of polymers can be aligned by streaming forces. Liquid crystals of this type seem to exist in cultured fibroblasts[39].

Last but not least the fibrocytes in tissue are also directly involved by their mechanical activity in the architectural organization of the polymers. When cultured within a tri-dimensional floating gel of collagen fibres fibroblasts rapidly attach to the polymers and gather them close to their membranes. It results in a progressive retraction of the lattice that can be inhibited by colchicine and cytochalasin B[40]. If the floating gel is immobilized between two captors, the network of fibres and the cells are oriented in a direction parallel to the developing force (Figure 18.10). After a few hours the traction developed by the fibrocytes is in the order of dgram per million cells[41]. Skin fibroblasts isolated from dermatosparactic calves or sheep are defective in this property of retraction[42]. The skin in these animals is very fragile and the network of fibrils is not organized in bundles[43]. These observations support the concept that the lateral packing of the fibrils in bundles and perhaps the spatial organization of the bundles is significantly determined by the resident fibrocytes. It has to be noted that similar defects in the mechanical properties of the fibroblasts do not occur in the Ehlers-Danlos syndrome including the type VII form, a disease in the human similar to dermatosparaxis biochemically, i.e. there is an increased concentration of the collagen precursor[44].

172

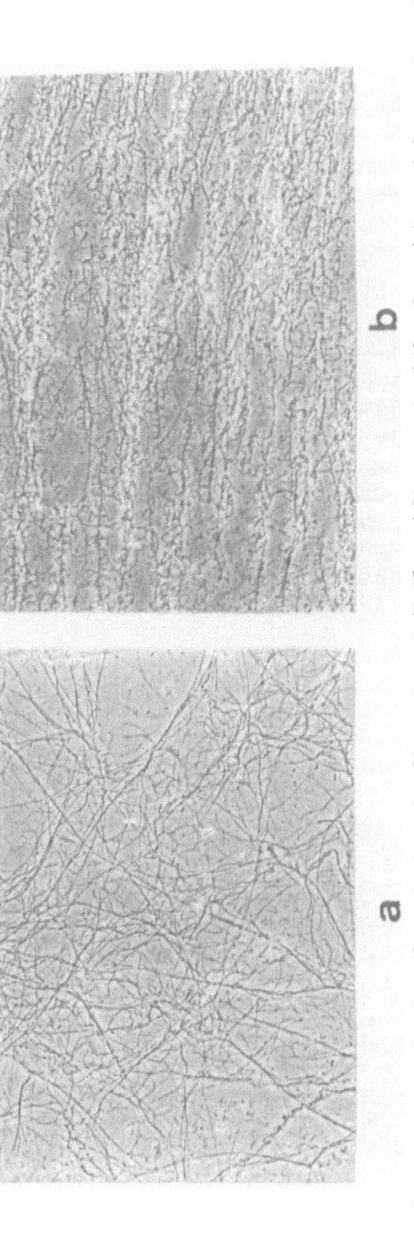

Figure 18.9 Heat polymerization of a solution of collagen type I (0.15 mg/ml) on an immobile plate (a) or shaken at 50 cycles per minute (b). Note the orientation of the polymers in the direction of the movement in (b). Phase contrast microscopy x 600

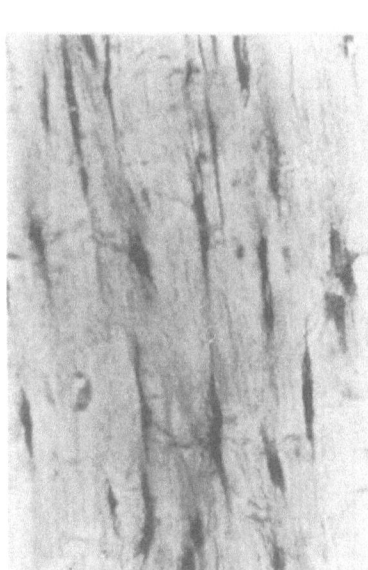

Figure 18.10 Immunoperoxidase localization of fibronectin around fibroblasts cultured within an immobilized collagen lattice. The cells and their surrounding coat of fibronectin are oriented in the direction of the collagen fibres stretched between the captors at the left and right sides of the gel x 800

173

In the floating collagen lattice the fibroblasts undergo a process of differentiation towards the phenotype of a dermal fibrocyte. They stop dividing, acquire different membrane permeability and modify their biosynthetic activity[45]. The repressed synthesis of collagen observed in floating gel does not occur in gels maintained under traction indicating that mechanical information is transferred to the cells by the support[46]. Such a mechanism might operate in vivo and be responsible for hypertrophy in scars under tension, for the increased thickness of the wall of arteries during hypertension and for the greater thickness of the dermis in the extensor than in the flexor side of joints.

CONCLUSIONS

The complex rheological properties of the dermis depend on the differentiated function of the fibrocytes. These cells synthesize the macromolecules that are the building blocks of a network displaying physical properties that will provide resistance to traction and compression and allow the diffusion of nutrients from and to the bloodstream. The plasticity of the network is made possible by a perfectly adapted architectural organization of the polymers that depends on the nature of the macromolecules, the function of the cells and their response to mechanical and other environmental stimuli. Both properties are required to allow the connective tissue to play its role of support.

REFERENCES

1. Pierard, G.E. and Lapière, Ch.M. (1981). Structure et fonctions du derme et de l'hypoderme. In Prunieras, M. (ed.) Précis de cosmétologie dermatolgoique. pp 37-50 (Paris: Masson)
2. Pierard, G.E. and Lapière, Ch.M. (1977). Physiopathological variations in the mechanical properties of skin. Arch. Dermatol. Res., 260, 231-9
3. Holbrook, K.A., Byers, P.H. and Pinnel, S.R. (1982). The structure and function of dermal connective tissue in normal individuals and patients with inherited connective tissue disorders. Scan. Electr. Micr., 4, 1731-44
4. Costa-Pereira, G., Guerra, F. and Bittencourt-Sampaio, S. (1976). Oxytalan, elaunin, and elastic fibres in the human skin. J. Invest. Dermatol., 66, 143-8
5. Pierard, G.E. (1986). How is the basement membrane attached to the dermis? Stereology of the interlacing fibers at the underface of the dermo-epidermal basement membrane. Am. J. Dermatopathol., 8, 234-6
6. Pierard, G.E. (1984). Structure et propriétées méchaniques des compartiments adventitiel et réticulaire du derme. PhD Thesis, Liège
7. Carton, R.W., Dainauskas, J. and Clark, J.W. (1962). Elastic properties of single elastic fibers. J. Appl. Physiol., 17, 547-51
8. Hall, D.A. (1971). The structure of elastin fibers. In Elden, H.R. (ed.) Biophysical Properties of the Skin. pp 187-218. (New York: Wiley-Interscience)
9. Mukkerjee, D. and Hoffman, A. (1971). Physical and mechanical properties of elastin. In Elden, H.R. (ed.) Biophysical Properties of the Skin. pp 219-41. (New York: Wiley-Interscience)
10. Stromberg, D.D. and Wiederhielm, C.A. (1969). Viscoelastic description of a collagenous tissue in simple elongation. J. Appl. Physiol., 26, 857-62
11. Burgeson, R.E. (1982). Genetic heterogeneity of collagens. J. Invest. Dermatol., 79, 255-305
12. Cleary, E.G. and Gibson, M.A. (1983). Elastin associated microfibrils and microfibrillar proteins. In Hall, D.A. and Jackson, D.S. (eds.) International Review of Connective Tissue Research. Vol.10, pp 97-209, (New York, London: Academic Press)

13. Mosher, D.F. and Furcht, L.T. (1981). Fibronectin: review of its structure and possible functions. J. Invest. Dermatol., **77**, 175-80
14. Scott, J.E. (1984). The periphery of the developing collagen fibril. Quantitative relationships with dermatan sulphate and other surface associated species. Biochem. J., **218**, 229-33
15. Lories, V., David, G., Cassiman, J.J. and Van Den Berghe, H. (1986). Heparan sulfate proteoglycans of human lung fibroblasts. Occurence of distinct membrane, matrix and secreted forms. Eur. J. Biochem., **158**, 351-360
16. Lenaers, A., Ansay, M., Nusgens, B. and Lapiere, Ch.M. (1971). Collagen made of extended alpha chains, procollagen, in genetically defective dermatosparaxic calves. Eur. J. Biochem., **23**, 533-43
17. Epstein, E.H. (1974). Alpha 1 (III) 3 human skin collagen. Release by pepsin digestion and preponderance in fetal life. J. Biol. Chem., **249**, 3225-31
18. Lapière, Ch.M., Nusgens, B., Pierard, G.E. and Hermanns, J.F. (1975). The involvement of procollagen in spatially orientated fibrogenesis. In Burleigh, P.M.C. and Poole, A.R. (eds.) Dynamics of Connective Tissue Macromolecules. pp 33-50. (Amsterdam: North-Holland Company)
19. Zimmermann, D.R., Trueb, B., Winterhalter, K.H., Witmer, R. and Fischer, R.W. (1986). Type VI collagen is a major component of the human cornea. FEBS Lett., **197**, 55-8
20. Weber, L., Kirsch, E., Muller, P. and Krieg, T. (1984). Collagen type distribution and macromolecular organization of connective tissue in different layers of the human skin. J. Invest. Dermatol., **82**, 156-60
21. Meigel, W.N., Gay, St. and Weber, L. (1977). Dermal architecture and collagen type distribution. Arch. Derm. Res., **259**, 1-10
22. Holbrook, K.A. and Byers, P.H. (1981). Ultrastructural characteristics of the skin in a form of the Ehlers-Danlos syndrome type IV: storage in the rough endoplasmic reticulum. Lab. Invest., **44**, 342-50
23. Burgeson, R.E., Morris, N.P., Murray, L.W., Duncan, K.G., Keene, D.R. and Sakai, L.Y. (1985). The structure of type VII collagen. In Fleischmajer, R., Olsen, B.R. and Kuhn, K. (eds.) Biology, Chemistry and Pathology of Collagen. Vol. 460, pp 47-57. (Ann. N.Y. Acad. Sci.)
24. Adachi, E. and Hayashi, T. (1985). In vitro formation of fine fibrils with a D-periodic banding pattern from type V collagen. Coll. Rel. Res., **5**, 225
25. Sandberg, L.B., Soskel, N.T. and Leslie, J.G. (1981). Elastin structure, biosythesis and relation to disease states. N. Engl. J. Med., **304**, 566-79
26. Pierard, G.E. (1983). Syndrome d'Ascher et Cutis Laxa. Ann. Derm. Vener., **110**, 237-40
27. Pierard, G.E., Pierard-Franchimont, C. and Lapière, Ch.M. (1983). Histopathological aid at the diagnosis of the Ehlers-Danlos syndrome, gravis and mitis types. Int. J. Dermatol., **22**, 300-4
28. Comper, W.D. and Laurent, T.C. (1978). Physiological function of connective tissue polysaccharides. Physiol. Rev., **58**, 255
29. Scott, J.E. and Haigh, M. (1985). Proteoglycan type I collagen fibril interactions in bone and non calcifying connective tissues. Biosci. Rep., **5**, 71-81
30. Woods, A., Couchman, J.R. and Hook, M. (1985). Heparan sulfate proteoglycans of rat embryo fibroblasts. A hydrophobic form may link cytoskeleton and matrix components. J. Biol. Chem., **260**, 10872-9
31. Nusgens, B., Merrill, C., Lapière, Ch.M. and Bell, E. (1984). Collagen biosynthesis by cells in a tissue equivalent matrix in vitro. Coll. Rel. Res., **4**, 351-64
32. Lapière, Ch.M. and Nusgens, B. (1974). Polymerization of procollagen in vitro. Biochem. Biophys. Acta, **342**, 237-46
33. Miyahara, M., Yayashi, K., Berger, J., Tanzawa, K., Njieha, F., Trelstad, R.L. and Prockop, D.J. (1984). Formation of collagen fibrils by enzyme cleavage of precursors of type I collagen in vitro. J. Biol. Chem., **259**, 9891-8
34. Trelstad, R.L., Hayashi, K. and Toole, B.P. (1974). Epithelial collagens and glycosaminoglycans in the embryonic cornea. Macromolecular order and morphogenesis in the basement membrane. J. Cell. Biol., **62**, 815-30
35. Lapière, Ch.M., Nusgens, B. and Pierard, G.E. (1977). Interaction between collagen type I and type III in conditioning bundles organization . Conn. Tissue. Res., **5**, 21-9
36. Trelstad, R.L. (1977). Mesenchymal cell polarity and morphogenesis of chick cartilage. Dev. Biol., **59**, 153-63
37. Trelstad, R.L. and Hayashi, K. (1979). Tendon collagen fibrillogenesis: intracellular subassemblies and cell surface changes associated with fibril growth. Dev. Biol., **71**, 228-42
38. Lapière, Ch.M., Nusgens, B., Pierard, G.E. and Hermanns, J.F. (1975). The involvement of procollagen in spatially orientated fibrogenesis. In Burleigh, M. and Poole, R. (eds.) Dynamics of Connective Tissues Macromolecules. pp 33-50. (Amsterdam: North Holland Publ. Co.)

39. Bruns, R.R., Hulmes, D.J.S., Therrien, S.F. and Gross, J. (1979). Procollagen segment-long-spacing (SLS) crystallites: their role in collagen fibrillogenesis. Proc. Natl. Acad. Sci. USA, **76**, 313-17

40. Bell, E., Ivarsson, B. and Merrill, C. (1979). Production of a tissue like structure by contraction of collagen lattices by human fibroblasts of different proliferative potential in vitro. Proc. Natl. Acad. Sci. USA, **76**, 1274-8

41. Delvoye, P., Leveque, J.L. and Lapière, Ch.M. (1986). Mechanical forces are developed by fibroblasts in a three-dimensional collagen lattice. J. Invest. Dermatol., (abstract), **87**, 135

42. Delvoye, P., Nusgens, B. and Lapière, Ch.M. (1983). The capacity of retracting a collagen matrix is lost by dermatosparactic skin fibroblasts. J. Invest. Dermatol., **81**, 267-70

43. Pierard, G.E. and Lapière, Ch.M. (1976). Skin in dermatosparaxis. Dermal microarchitecture and biomechanical properties. J. Invest. Dermatol., **66**, 2-7

44. Delvoye, P., Mauch, C., Krieg, T. and Lapière, Ch.M. (1986). Contraction of collagen lattices by fibroblasts from patients and animals with heritable disorders of connective tissue. Br. J. Dermatol., **115**, 139-46

45. Bell, E., Sher, S., Hull, B., Merrill, C., Rosen, S., Chamson, A., Asselineud, D., Dubertret, L., Coulomb, B., Lapière, Ch.M., Nusgens, B. and Neveux, Y. (1983). The reconstitution of living skin. J. Invest. Dermatol., **81**, 2S-10S

46. Delvoye, P., Dreze, S., Nusgens, B. and Lapière, Ch.M. (1986). Mechanical regulation of collagen biosynthesis, FECTS meeting, Manchester, 25-31 July 1986, Abstract no. 169

Section VI

PHYSICAL PROPERTIES

Chapter 19

Optical properties of skin: measurement of erythema

B L Diffey

Optical radiation incident on the skin may be: reflected at the skin surface due to a change in refractive index between air and stratum corneum; absorbed by chromophores in the epidermis or dermis; scattered by cell organelles in the epidermis or collagen in the dermis; or transmitted to deeper tissues. The reflection of light from the surface of the skin is always between 4% and 7% for both black and white skin[1]. Ultraviolet radiation (UVR) and visible light that enters the skin will be scattered mainly in a forward direction in the epidermis[2] due to Mie scattering by cell organelles, e.g. melanosomes, which have dimensions of the order of the wavelength of light[3]. In the dermis, however, scattering is much more isotropic and light re-emitted from skin in vivo comes largely from the dermis[4]. Dermal scattering increases rapidly with decreasing wavelength in an approximate manner predicted by Rayleigh scattering in which the probability of scattering varies inversely with the fourth power of the wavelength. Consequently, dermal scattering determines principally the depth to which different wavelengths of optical radiation penetrate the dermis.

The penetration of optical radiation of different wavelengths into the skin is illustrated schematically in Figure 19.1. The major chromophores which determine the depth of penetration in the different spectral regions are summarized in Table 19.1.

Table 19.1 Cutaneous chromophores for optical radiation

Spectral region	Wavelength interval (nm)	Major chromophores	
		Epidermis	Dermis
UV-C	200-290	Nucleic acids Aromatic amino acids	
UV-B	290-320	Melanin	
UV-A	320-400	Melanin	
Blue light	400-500	Melanin	Haemoglobin Bilirubin β-carotene
Green light	500-570	Melanin	Haemoglobin
Red light	570-760	Melanin	

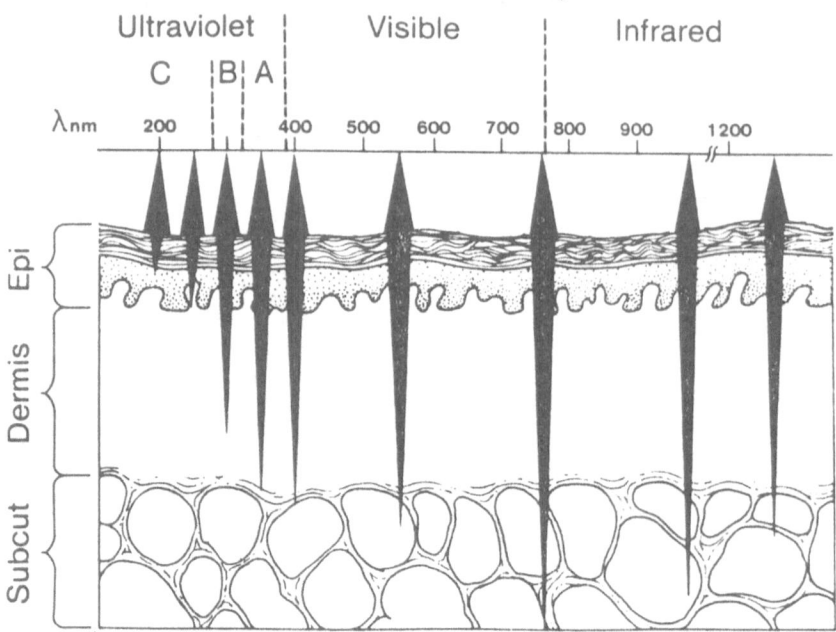

Figure 19.1 A diagrammatic summary of the penetration of optical radiation of different wavelengths into human skin

MEASUREMENT OF ERYTHEMA

Erythema induced by ultraviolet radiation or other external stimuli results in increased blood content of the subpapillary vascular plexus. When this happens a greater amount of blue and green light is absorbed and less is reflected. In contrast, the amount of red light absorbed or reflected shows little change with vasodilation. Hence the erythematous sites appear red to the eye by a process of subtractive colour mixing. The remainder of this chapter will describe five techniques based on the optical properties of the skin that have been used to attempt to quantify cutaneous erythema.

VISUAL SCALES

The human eye/brain system has been the most common means of assessing erythema. In studies of the effect of ultraviolet radiation and other stimuli on the skin, most of the interpretations have been based on an ordinal scale as illustrated in Table 19.2. There are several drawbacks to this type of rating scale[5]. Firstly, there is the danger that linearity will be assumed where none exists or where none has been established. Secondly, the visual detection of erythema is subjective and is affected by several unrelated factors such as viewing geometry, ambient illumination, and colour of unexposed surrounding skin. Also the experience and visual acuity of the observer can affect the score he attributes to each erythematous site.

Since the eye is much more suited to discriminating colour than quantifying the degree of colour, the dose of stimulus (UVR, chemical) that produces a minimal erythema has most often been the index chosen for semiquantitative evaluation of erythema. But even here, different definitions of the so-called 'minimal erythema dose' (MED) are adopted by different workers[6] so leaving some room for misunderstanding.

Table 19.2 Convention for grading of skin erythema (from ref.6)

Symbol	Abbreviation	Definition
0	NR	No reaction; identical to surrounding non-irradiated skin
±	MPE	Minimal perceptible erythema; blotchy areas of faint erythema confined to the irradiated site; borders indefinite
+	1+	Minimal erythema with four sharp borders
++	2+	More pronounced erythema without oedema
+++	3+	Marked erythema with oedema
++++	4+	Violaceous erythema with vesiculation

COLOUR COMPARISON CHART

The grading of the degree of erythema by using red-coloured papers as standards of comparison was first carried out by Hausser and Vahle in 1927[7]. These workers made a series of red-coloured solutions of different dilutions, which were put onto matt skin-coloured paper. The object is to match the erythematous site with the appropriate hue of red. This is theoretically a much sounder system than the visual rating scale since errors in colour perception can be obviated to some degree by using the eye as a null system - something it is good at. The main drawback of this system is that the colour standards do not have the general appearance of skin in that they lack the details of hairs, surface texture, translucency and irregularities of colour which are conspicuous on visual examination.

RED-COLOURED OPTICAL FILTERS

An alternative to using red-coloured paper is to interpose a series of pale, red-tinted gelatin filters between the eye and the erythematous site[8]. The degree of redness is estimated by noting which red filter just causes the erythema to disappear. The series of filters should have a high transmittance for red light ($\lambda > 600$ nm) with decreasing transmittance for blue-green light. The series of red filters should be arranged so that there is a constant fractional difference in absorbance of blue-green light between the successive filters. It is also important that the spectrum of the light source used for inspecting the skin should be continuous in the visible region with ample quantities of red light; sunlight and tungsten lamps are a good choice, but cool white fluorescent lamps are a poor choice since they emit little red light.

REFLECTANCE SPECTROPHOTOMETRY

The principle of this technique is to measure the reflectance of light of different wavelengths from the skin. Complete reflectance spectra over the ultraviolet and visible regions require a spectrophotometer which is both bulky and expensive. Such sophisticated equipment is unnecessary for quantifying erythema because if we examine the reflectance spectra of normal and erythematous skin (Figure 19.2), we can see that there is a reduction in the reflectance of green light (around 550 nm) from the erythematous skin. In fact, the reason our skin looks red when we get sunburnt is not because more red light is reflected from the skin, but rather that less green light is reflected. Instruments for quantifying erythema by measuring the amount of green light re-emitted from the skin in vivo were first developed in the 1950s and 1960s[9]. Since these early days there have been considerable advances in electro-optical technology resulting in the construction of instruments which are easier to use and more reliable[10].

The principle of operation of the instrument shown in Figure 19.3 compares the amount of reflected red and green light and obtains an 'erythema index' which is evaluated electronically as:

$$\log_{10}\left(\frac{\text{Intensity of red component of reflected light}}{\text{Intensity of green component of reflected light}}\right)$$

The white light from a projector bulb is focused on to the aperture of one branch of a trifurcated fibre optic cable. The common leg of the fibre optic cable is supported 1 mm from the skin surface in a conically-shaped applicator. Light re-emitted from the skin passes up the other two branches; one of these is optically coupled to a green interference filter and photodiode, and the other is optically coupled to a red interference filter and photodiode. The photocurrents from both photodiodes are amplified and form the two inputs to a log ratio module. The output from this module is displayed as the erythema index. An external zero control adjusts the gain of one of the amplifiers such that when the applicator attached to the common leg of the fibre optic cable is in contact with a white diffuse reflectance plaque, both inputs to the log ratio

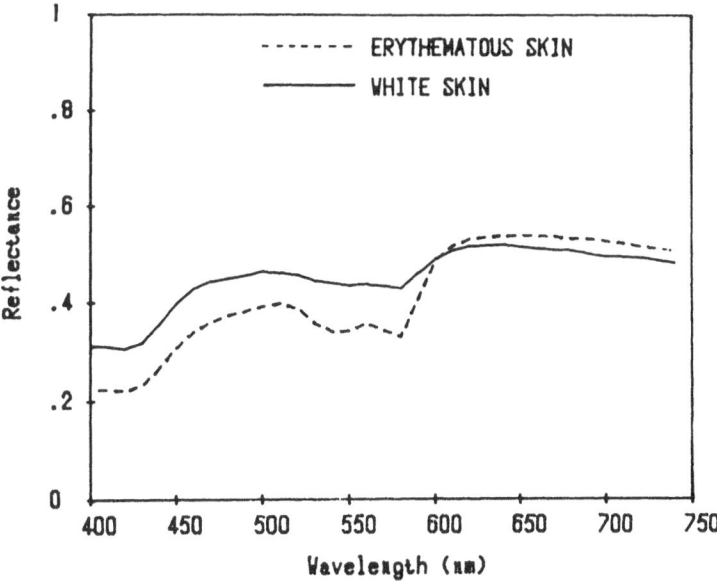

Figure 19.2 The reflectance spectra of normal and erythematous Caucasian skin in vivo

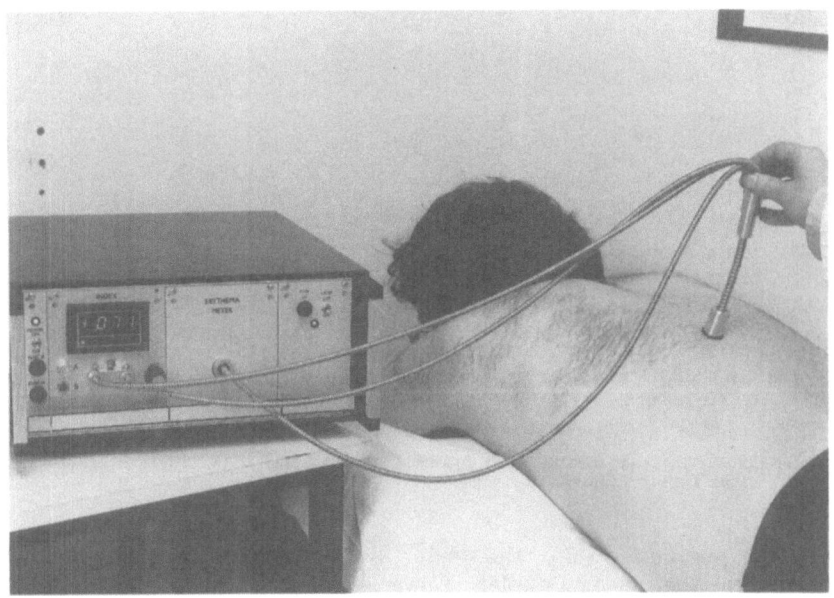

Figure 19.3 The measurement of erythema on the back of a subject using a reflectance instrument (from ref. 11)

module are made equal, resulting in a displayed erythema index of zero. The instrument may be used in normal room lighting.

This instrument is more sensitive than the eye at detecting 'redness'. It will record an increase in erythema index at an irradiated skin site in which there appears to be no visible erythema[11] and can detect red pigment in solutions at dilutions approximately one order of magnitude higher than were detected by eye[10].

LASER DOPPLER VELOCIMETRY

When light is scattered from skin, a proportion of the light will have been scattered from static structures within the skin and a portion from moving red cells. The light scattered from the moving red cells will be at a slightly different frequency, or wavelength, from the incident light due to an effect known as the Doppler effect.

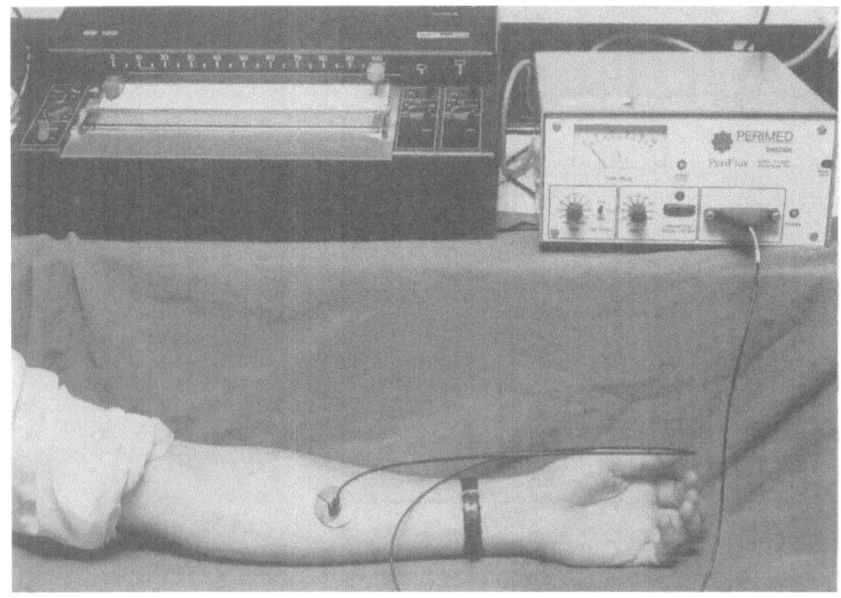

Figure 19.4 The measurement of blood cell flux on the volar forearm of a subject using a laser Doppler flowmeter

The frequency of the red He-Ne laser used as the light source in the laser Doppler flowmeter shown in Figure 19.4 is 4.7×10^{14} Hz, and after scattering from blood cells moving at a typical velocity of 1 mm/s, a frequency shift of about 3 kHz is produced. The mixture of scattered light travelling back up the fibre optic to the photodetector gives rise to electrical signals produced by the photodetector which have a frequency characteristic of the Doppler shifted frequency[12]. So the faster the red cells are moving, the greater will be the Doppler shifted frequency. And the more red cells there are in the field of view of the probe tip, the greater will be the intensity of red light scattered from the skin and the stronger the electrical signal produced by the photodetector. The instrument then displays a needle deflection which is proportional to the blood cell flux. This is defined as the number of red blood cells moving in the measured volume multiplied by the mean cell velocity. However, the signal produced from a laser Doppler flowmeter is time-varying (Figure 19.5). There is a slow frequency component (0.1-0.2 Hz) thought to be dependent on vasomotor tone, and a fast frequency oscillation attributable to the pulsatile nature of blood flow. Most instruments incorporate a long time constant on the ratemeter to smoothe out these oscillations, although it is probably better to record the time varying signal on a chart recorder and estimate the mean deflection by eye.

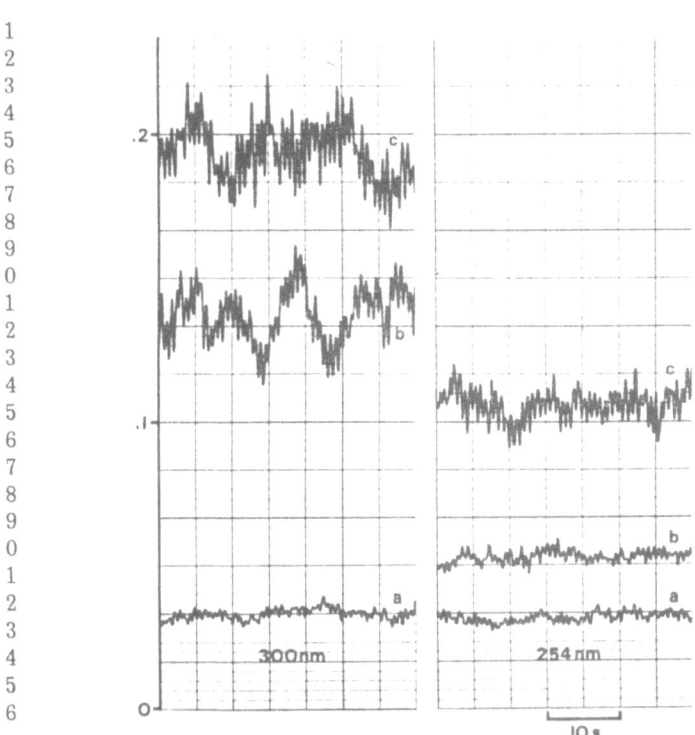

Figure 19.5 The recording obtained with a laser Doppler flowmeter 24 h after exposure to different doses of UVB and UVC radiation (curves b and c). Curve 'a' is an unirradiated site

COMPARISON OF ULTRAVIOLET DOSE-ERYTHEMAL RESPONSE CURVES

Examples of ultraviolet dose-erythemal response curves measured using each of the five techniques described above are shown in Figure 19.6.

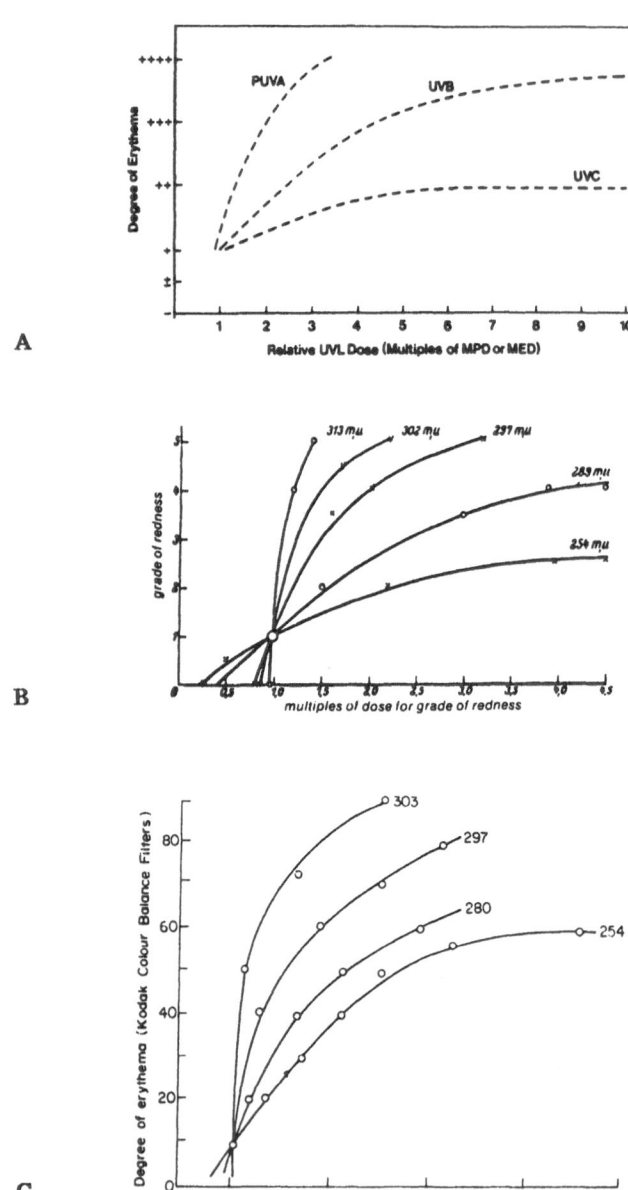

Dose-response curves obtained using visual scales for UVC radiation, UVB radiation and psoralen-UVA (PUVA) are little more than qualitative (Figure 19.6A). Note that there are not even any data points. Figures 19.6B and 19.6C present dose-response curves for different wavelengths of UVR obtained using coloured papers[7] and red-coloured filters[13], respectively. Both these examples of

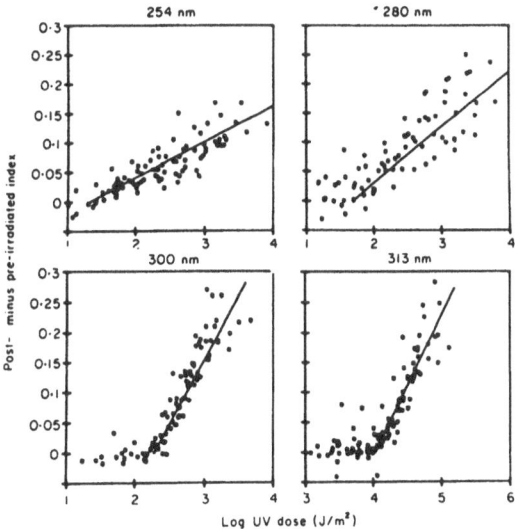

D

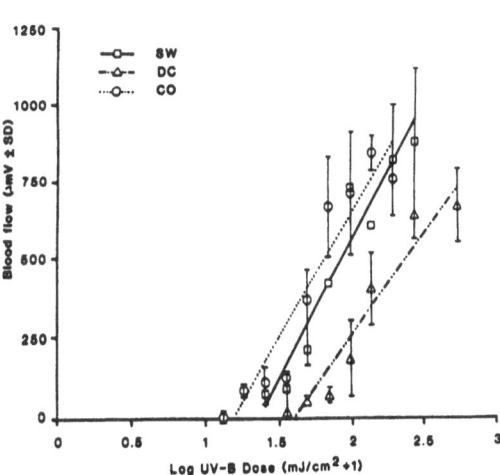

E

Figure 19.6 Example of ultraviolet dose-erythemal response curves determined by the five different techniques. A = visual scales[16]; B = coloured papers[7]; C = red-coloured filters[13]; D = reflectance instrument[14]; E = laser Doppler flowmeter[15]

dose-response curves show essentially the same information; in particular, that erythema increases more rapidly with multiples of the MED for UVR of around 300 nm (UVB) than for 254 nm radiation (UVC). These techniques are only semiquantitative in that they both rely upon a subjective colour matching by the observer. Pooled dose-response curves obtained on a total of 38 Caucasian subjects for four different wavelengths of UVR obtained by a reflectance instrument[10] are shown in Figure 19.6D. In this case, the logarithm of UV dose has been plotted along the abscissa, and at doses in excess of the least dose of UVR to result in visible erythema, an approximate linear response is obtained[14]. The slope of the linear part of the dose-response curve was considerably higher for wavelengths of 300 and 313 nm than for 254 nm, confirming the impressions obtained by earlier workers (Figures 19.6B and 19.6C). Finally, Figure 19.6E shows the dose-response curves in three subjects obtained at 24 h after UVB irradiation and measured using a laser Doppler flowmeter[15].

CONCLUSION

Visual scales for assessing erythema are entirely subjective; coloured papers and red-coloured filters depend upon the lighting conditions and observer's visual acuity as well as degree of erythema; reflectance instruments and laser Doppler flowmeters are objective methods of measuring erythema.

REFERENCES

1. Anderson, R.R. and Parrish, J.A. (1981). The optics of human skin. J. Invest. Dermatol., **77**, 13-19
2. Bruls, W.A.G. and van der Leun, J.C. (1984). Forward scattering properties of human epidermal layers. Photochem. Photobiol. **40**, 231-42
3. Diffey, B.L. (1983). A mathematical model for ultraviolet optics in skin. Phys. Med. Biol., **28**, 647-57
4. Anderson, R.R., Hu, J. and Parrish, J.A. (1981). Optical radiation transfer in the human skin and applications in vivo remittance spectroscopy. In Marks, R. and Payne, P.A. (eds.) Bioengineering and the Skin. p 243. (Lancaster: MTP Press Ltd)
5. Daniels, F. and Imbrie, J.D. (1958). Comparison between visual grading and reflectance measurements of erythema produced by sunlight. J. Invest. Dermatol., **30**, 295-304
6. Hawk, J.L.M. and Parrish, J.A. (1982). Responses of normal skin to ultraviolet radiation. In Regan, J.D. and Parrish, J.A. (eds.) The Science of Photomedicine. pp 219-60. (New York: Plenum Press)
7. Hausser, K.W. and Vahle, W. (1927). Sonnerbrand und Sonnenbraunung. Wissenschaftliche Veroffnungen des Siemens Konzern, **6**, 101-20
8. Argenbright, L.W. and Forbes, P.D. (1982). Erythema and skin blood content. Br. J. Dermatol., **106**, 569-74
9. Tronnier, H. (1969). Evaluation and measurement of ultraviolet erythema. In Urbach, F. (ed.) The Biologic Effects of Ultraviolet Radiation with Emphasis on the Skin. p 255. (Oxford: Pergammon Press)
10. Diffey, B.L., Oliver, R.J. and Farr, P.M. (1984). A portable instrument for quantifying erythema induced by ultraviolet radiation. Br. J. Dermatol., **111**, 663-72
11. Farr, P.M. and Diffey, B.L. (1984). Quantitative studies on cutaneous erythema induced by ultraviolet radiation. Br. J. Dermatol., **111**, 673-82
12. Nilsson, G.E., Tenland, T. and Oberg, P.A. (1980). Evaluation of a laser Doppler flowmeter for measurement of tissue blood flow. IEEE Trans. Biomed. Eng., **BME-27**, 597-604

13. Berger, D., Urbach, F. and Davies, R.E. (1968). The action spectrum of erythema induced by ultraviolet radiation. Preliminary report. In Jadassohn, W. and Schirren, C.G. (eds.) XIII Congressus Internationalis Dermatologiae. p 1112. (Berlin: Springer)
14. Farr, P.M. and Diffey, B.L. (1985). The erythemal response of human skin to ultraviolet radiation. Br. J. Dermatol., 113, 65-76
15. Young, A.R., Guy, R.H. and Maibach, H.I. (1985). Laser Doppler velocimetry to quantify UV-B induced increase in human skin blood flow. Photochem. Photobiol., 42, 385-90
16. Parrish, J.A., Stern, R.S., Pathak, M.A. and Fitzpatrick, T.B. (1982). Photochemotherapy of skin diseases. In Regan, J.D. and Parrish, J.A. (eds.) The Science of Photomedicine. p 595-623. (New York: Plenum Press)

Chapter 20

The thermal properties of skin

J C Barbenel

INTRODUCTION

Heat is produced by metabolic processes within the cells of the body. As a consequence the body, and particularly its core, is generally at a higher temperature than the surrounding environment. Because of this temperature difference, there is a flow of heat from the body to the surroundings, the terminal part of this process being heat transfer across the skin. The skin has a large surface area, and heat loss via the skin, and the modification of this heat transfer in response to environmental conditions, is of great importance in maintaining body temperature within the narrow limits which are required for normal cellular function.

The transfer of heat across the skin involves two basic mechanisms. The first of these is conductive heat transfer, entirely analogous to the heat conduction which occurs in passive materials such as metal. In addition, the flowing blood can carry heat - a process known as convective transfer.

The rate of heat transfer depends on the temperature gradients in the body, but also on the thermal properties of the tissues, although which properties are of primary importance depends on the heat transfer conditions.

PASSIVE HEAT TRANSFER

The thermal parameters which determine conductive heat transfer rates depend on whether the heat transfer is in a steady-state or equilibrium, or is changing due to some alteration which peturbs the thermal equilibrium of the system, e.g. a change in the environmental temperature.

Steady-state or equilibrium heat flow

Under steady-state conditions, the temperature of the material through which the heat transfers remains constant. Hence all the heat entering is conducted through the material (Figure 20.1).

Assuming that the skin can be considered as thermally homogeneous and that the heat flows in one direction, the heat flux, or rate of heat flow (H) per unit area (A) normal to the direction of flow is proportional to the temperature gradient (dT/dx) or:

$$\frac{H}{A} \propto \frac{dT}{dx} \qquad (1)$$

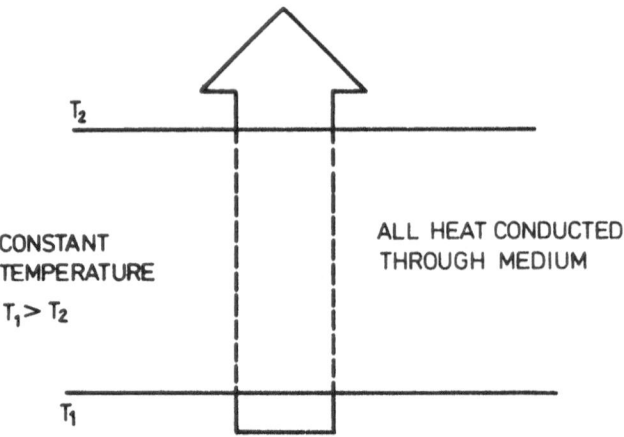

T_2

CONSTANT
TEMPERATURE

$T_1 > T_2$

ALL HEAT CONDUCTED
THROUGH MEDIUM

T_1

Figure 20.1 Under steady-state conditions all the heat entering the medium is conducted through it

which may be re-written as:

$$H = kA\frac{dT}{dx} \qquad (2)$$

The constant of proportionality, k, is known as the thermal conductivity. The SI unit is $W\ m^{-1}\ K^{-1}$ but values are widely quoted in $cal\ cm^{-1}\ s^{-1}\ {}^{\circ}C^{-1}$ ($1\ cal\ cm^{-1}\ s^{-1}\ {}^{\circ}C^{-1} = 418.7\ W\ m^{-1}\ K^{-1}$). When the numerical value of thermal conductivity is high, the material is a good conductor, and the heat flow produced by a given temperature gradient is high. Inversely, if it is low the material is a poor conductor or an insulator, and the heat flow for the same temperature gradient is small.

Two cases in which the geometry of the tissues can be simplified are of special interest.

In areas of skin which can be considered as being flat, and having the geometry shown in Figure 20.2 then the rate of heat flow across it is given by:

$$H = \frac{kA(T_2 - T_1)}{d} \qquad (3)$$

Some areas of the body, such as the arm, may be considered as approximately cylindrical (Figure 20.3). For a length L of the cylinder with inner radius a, at the temperature T_a, and outer radius b, at temperature T_b, the rate of heat flow is given by:

$$H = \frac{2kL(T_a - T_b)}{\ln(b/a)} \qquad (4)$$

192

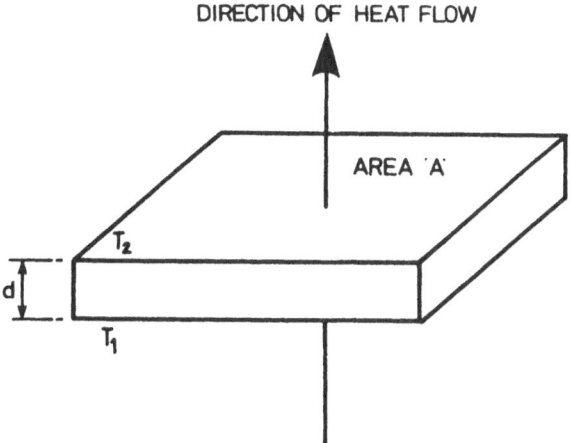

Figure 20.2 Steady-state heat flow in a rectangular block

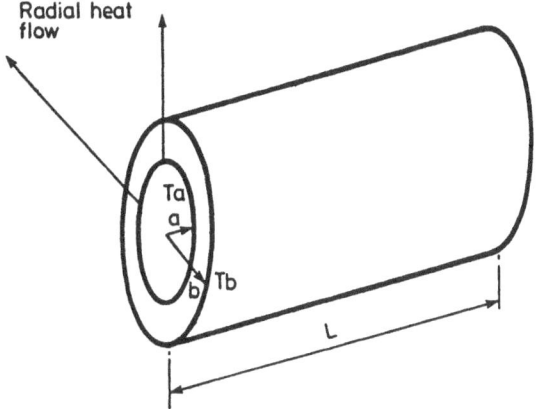

Figure 20.3 Steady-state heat flow in a cylinder

Transient heat flow

The steady-state heat flow described in the previous section will be disrupted if there is any alteration in the thermal conditions, e.g. an increase in the skin surface temperature. This will result in a change in the temperature distribution and an increase in the temperature throughout the depth of the skin, a change which requires a supply of heat. Thus not all the heat entering the skin will be conducted through the tissue, some will be stored as the altered skin temperature (Figure 20.4). Under these conditions, two additional thermal parameters become important in addition to the thermal conductivity. The specific heat capacity (c, units $J kg^{-1} K^{-1}$) of the material is the amount of heat required to raise the temperature of unit mass by 1 K or 1°C. The quantity of heat (Q) which must be supplied to a body of mass m, to raise the temperature through an interval ΔT is given by:

$$Q = mc\Delta T \tag{5}$$

The heat flow in equations 1-3 contains the thickness and area of tissue but equation (5) contains the mass. The other parameter which is important is the density (ρ, units $kg m^{-3}$) which provides a connection between the geometrical variables and the tissue mass.

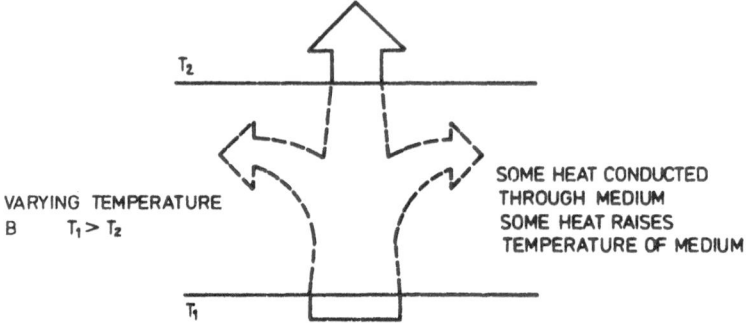

Figure 20.4 During transient heat flow not all the heat entering the medium is conducted through it

The temperature distribution in the skin after thermal equilibrium has been disturbed would depend on all three parameters, k, c and ρ, and will evolve with time. In general the mathematical description of the transient response is very much more complicated than the simple equations describing steady-state conditions.

Two transient solutions are of considerable practical importance. The first was derived by Buettner[1]. Irradiation of the skin surface will raise the temperature of that surface. The increase in skin surface temperature ΔT is proportional to the intensity of the radiation absorbed by the skin, I. The equation relating these variables is:

$$\Delta T = \frac{2I\sqrt{t}}{\sqrt{(\pi k\rho c)}} \tag{6}$$

The thermal equilibrium of the skin may also be disrupted by bringing a block of material at an initial temperature T_m into contact with the skin surface. Unlike the previous transient problem, this is entirely passive - no additional heat is added to the medium after initial contact. Under these conditions a new thermal equilibrium will be established after sufficient time has elapsed. If the block of material is large, it is possible to determine this equilibrium contact temperature, T_c, by calculating the relevant heat balance equations[2,3],

$$\frac{(T_s - T_c)}{(T_c - T_m)} = \frac{\sqrt{(k\rho c)_m}}{\sqrt{(k\rho c)_s}} \qquad (7)$$

or,

$$T_c = \frac{T_m\sqrt{(k\rho c)_m} + T_s\sqrt{(k\rho c)_s}}{\sqrt{(k\rho c)_m} + \sqrt{(k\rho c)_s}} \qquad (8)$$

Where $(k\rho c)_m$ refers to the thermal properties of the block, $(k\rho c)_s$ is that of the skin and T_s is the initial temperature of the skin surface.

In equations 6-8 the thermal parameters appear as the product $k\rho c$, a group which occurs in many solutions to transient heat flow problems. The physical meaning of the product can best be understood by considering equation 6, which implies that for a given value of radiation intensity, the temperature rise at the skin surface is dependent on $k\rho c$. The greater the numerical value of this product the smaller the temperature rise, and it is therefore known as the thermal inertia.

BLOOD FLOW

The blood supply to the tissues carries not only nutrients, it also conveys heat. Heat will be exchanged between the blood and tissues whenever there is a temperature difference, and this provides a route of transfer quite independent of, and different to, the conductive transfer discussed in the previous section. In general, the blood entering the skin is warmer than tissues and heat is therefore transmitted from the blood to the skin. The rate, and therefore the extent of this transfer, is ill understood. It is generally assumed in discussing this convective heat transfer that the rate of increase of heat in the tissues ($\dot{Q}$) is directionally proportional to the temperature difference between the blood (T_{ar}) and the tissue (T_t) and the rate of blood flow ($\dot{m}$). The rate of increase of heat gained by the tissues is given approximately by:

$$\dot{Q} = \dot{m}c_b(T_{ar} - T_t) \qquad (9)$$

Once again one of the thermal parameters, the specific heat of the blood c_b, appears in equation 9.

The heat balance in equation 9 is based on the assumption that complete thermal equilibrium is attained between blood and tissue. The justification for this assumption is by no means clear. Paterson[4] used previous analyses[5,6] to investigate the problem, and suggested that the extent of heat transfer depended on the group of variables, $L/(vd^2)$, where L is a characteristic length and d a characteristic diameter of the vessels involved, and v is the mean blood flow rate. He concluded that if the numerical value of the parameter was less than approximately 1.25×10^8 s m^{-2} complete thermal equilibrium would be attained. The values he calculated for capillaries suggested that heat exchange between the blood and the tissues would be complete, and that they would attain the same temperature.

The capillary blood supply in the skin is extremely complex, being made up of capillary loops reaching towards the dermal-epidermal junction and plexuses at both subcapillary and subdermal level[7]. The skin temperature, and the possible amount of heat transfer, differ at these different levels. The blood supply to the various levels can be modified and this gives a mechanism for controlling the heat transfer from the blood to the skin, and the heat loss across the skin.

MEASUREMENT OF THERMAL PROPERTIES

The thermal properties of the skin can be measured by excising tissue samples and carrying out controlled laboratory tests. The alternative technique of measuring either thermal inertia or the thermal conductivity of the skin in situ provides clinically more relevant information, which is, however, rather more difficult to interpret.

Thermal conductivity of excised tissue

The thermal conductivity of excised tissue samples can be determined by measuring the temperature gradient across the sample produced by a known heat flow. Henriques and Moritz[8] investigated the thermal conductivity of excised samples of porcine epidermis, dermis and subcutaneous fat and suggested values of 5×10^{-4}, 9×10^{-4} and 4×10^{-4} cal cm^{-1} s^{-1} °C^{-1} for the conductivity of these tissues. Hatfield and Pugh[9] used a similar method to determine the thermal conductivity of excised fat, obtaining a value of 4.9×10^{-4} cal cm^{-1} s^{-1} °C^{-1}. The relative values suggest a correlation with water content of the tissues and this has been confirmed by Spells[10] and Poppendiek et al.[11]. The thermal conductivity is an approximately linear function of the water content of the tissues considered for both fluids such as human blood and solids such as muscle and white matter.

Thermal inertia

The thermal inertia of the skin can be measured experimentally by irradiating the skin surface with a known intensity of irradiation and measuring the resulting skin surface temperature rise. The skin may first be blackened to improve the absorption. With excised skin there is a steady rise in skin temperature and, if the results are plotted in a form which is suggested by equation 6, there will be a linear relationship between the square of the temperature rise and a group involving the intensity and duration of irradiation (Figure 20.5). The irradiation of skin in situ produces rather different results. There is an initial linear temperature rise as predicted by theory, but the rate of temperature increase falls off to produce a relatively constant value of skin surface temperature elevation. The obliteration of blood flow in the skin removes this second phase of behaviour, which is almost certainly related to the response of the skin blood vessels to the increased temperature.

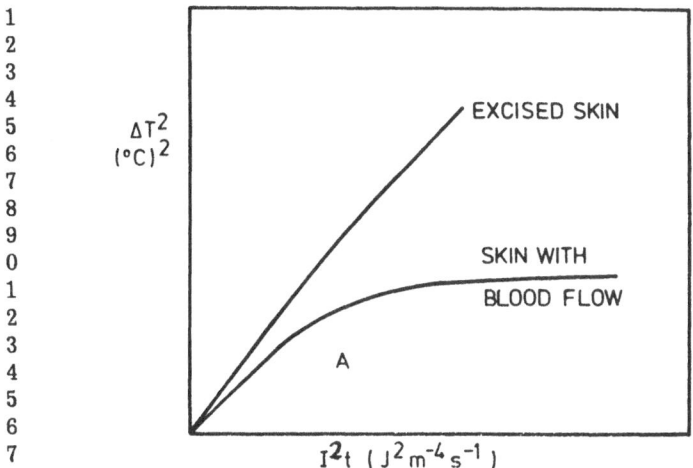

Figure 20.5 Irradiating the skin surface increases its temperature, but blood flow will influence the response

When the skin blood flow is intact the linear relationship occurs for the first 20 seconds or less[12], yielding a value for $k\rho c$ of 9×10^{-4} cal^2 cm^{-4} °C^{-2} s^{-1}. Thereafter the values reported vary from 9×10^{-4} cal^2 cm^{-4} °C^{-2} s^{-1} for skin with the blood supply occluded, to 5×10^{-3} cal^2 cm^{-4} °C^{-2} s^{-1} for skin in which the circulation was present. Buettner[1] produced a similar range of values, which depended on the state of vasodilatation.

In order to obtain the thermal conductivity from the thermal inertia it is necessary to know the value of the density and specific heat of the tissues. Stoll and Green[13], have suggested that the product of these two variables is very nearly equal to unity in cgs units (4186 in SI units), simplifying the calculation.

Thermal conductivity measurements in situ

Attempts have been made to adapt the laboratory methods to investigate thermal conductivity for in vivo use. Hensel and Bender[14] described a device for determining thermal conductivity in which the temperature difference between a series of heated and non-heated thermocouples, all applied to the skin surface, was measured (Figure 20.6). As with the irradiation method for determining the thermal inertia described above, the blood acts as a heat sink, and the main purpose of this and subsequent devices was the assessment of blood flow. There is little doubt that such devices do give an indication of changes in blood flow in the dermis, but there is at present no way of quantifying the output of such systems. Theoretical and experimental studies[15] suggest that, even under optimal conditions, the thermal effects due to the convective influence of blood flow is less than that due to tissue conduction. In addition, it is impossible to determine the route of the heat flow and thus the depth of tissue which is being sampled.

An interesting application of the principle may be the determination of the thermal conductivity and, hence, water content of the epidermis. In theory, the heat source and measurement point may be placed very closely together, when only the superficial tissues will be sampled (Figure 20.6). Unfortunately, in order to obtain reliable results, it is necessary that the thermal conductivity of the device itself be very much less than that of the epidermis. Difficulties in providing a suitable material, and the precision required in the construction, have so far limited the possible applications of such systems.

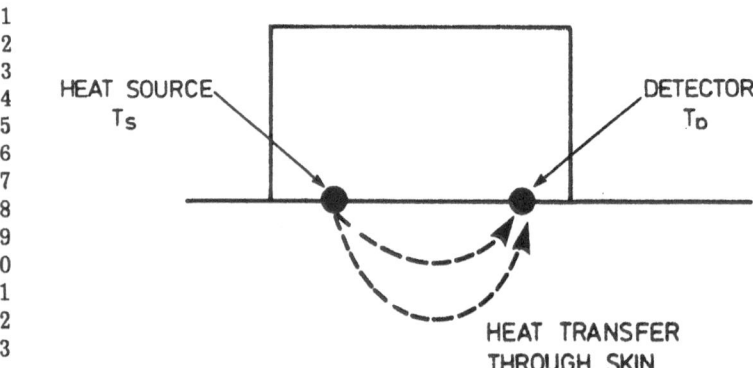

Figure 20.6 Heat is conducted from the heat source. The thermal conductivity of the skin is related to the difference in temperature between the source and detector

MATHEMATICAL MODELS OF HEAT TRANSFER THROUGH THE SKIN

By considering the conservation of energy, the general three-dimensional equation for heat transfer in perfused tissue can be obtained. The 'bio-heat' equation was first proposed by Pennes[16]:

$$\rho c \frac{\partial T}{\partial t} = k \nabla^2 T + \dot{m} c_b (T_{ar} - T) + \dot{Q} \qquad (10)$$

where T is the tissue temperature, t is time, $\dot{Q}$ the local metabolic rate per unit volume of tissue, and the other symbols are as previously defined. The first term on the right-hand side of equation 10 represents the conduction of heat through the tissues, and is a three-dimensional generalization of equation 1. The second term is the convective transfer of equation 9.

The derivation of equation 10 requires several major simplifying assumptions to be made. The most important are that the tissues can be considered as thermally homogeneous and isotropic and that the heat conduction and storage can be described by the general linear theory of heat transfer[17].

The use of equation 10 to obtain temperature-time profiles for the tissues is complicated. In general, there are three areas of difficulty. The first of these is the choice of how to represent the tissues. In the simplest case, the tissues can be represented as a single uniform layer, which may be rectangular, cylindrical or spherical. The mathematical simplicity of a single region is attractive, but the thermal effect of dermal blood flow cannot be adequately represented. This has given rise to multilayer models, the thermal and physiological properties of which may be discontinuous at the boundaries. There is also a major problem of how the dermal blood flow may be incorporated into the model. An interesting suggestion by Patterson[18], that it may be represented as a discontinuous heat source at the boundary between two layers, has been incorporated into a mathematical model of the superficial tissues[19] (this paper also gives details of alternative models). The third difficulty lies in the mathematical solution of the detailed model. Analytical methods have been used but numerical techniques, particularly finite difference methods, have been widely employed.

CONCLUSION

A knowledge of the thermal properties of the skin is of great importance in modelling heat transfer through the superficial tissues. In addition, the measurement of the thermal parameters may be important in describing the skin, and assessing the dermal blood flow. There are no universally agreed methods for in vivo measurement, nor are the meaning and interpretation of the experimental results understood. In this, as in so many other areas in the physical properties of skin, much work remains to be done.

REFERENCES

1. Buettner, R. (1936). The influence of blood circulation on the transport of heat in the skin. Strahlentherapie, **55**, 333
2. Myers, G.E. (1971). Analytical Methods in Conduction Heat Transfer. Ch 6, p 202. (New York: McGraw Hill)
3. Vendrik, A.J.H. and Vos, J.J.A. (1957). A method for the measurement of the thermal conductivity of the skin. J. Appl. Physiol., **11**, 211-15
4. Patterson, J. (1982). Heat and matter transfer in body organs with special reference to skin blood flow and localised hyperthermia. PhD Thesis, Bioengineering Unit, University of Strathclyde
5. Graetz, L. (1883). Uber die Warmeleitfahigkeit von Flussigkeiten. Ann. Phys. (N.F.), **18**, 79-94
6. Teorrel, L.M. and Nilsson, S.K. (1978). Temperature gradients in low flow vessels. Phys. Med. Biol., **23**, 106-17
7. Spaltholz, W. (1927). Blutegefasse der Haut Hand der Haut und Geschlechskraukh. Vol. 1, p 379. (Berlin: Springer)
8. Henriques, F.C. and Moritz, A.R. (1947). Studies of thermal injury. I. The conduction of heat to and through skin and the temperatures attained therein. A theoretical and an experimental investigation. Am. J. Pathol., **23**, 531-49
9. Hatfield, H.S. and Pugh, L.G.C. (1951). Thermal conductivity of human fat and muscle. Nature (Lond.), **168**, 918-19
10. Spells, K.E. (1960). The thermal conductivities of some biological fluids. Phys. Med. Biol., **5**, 139-53
11. Poppendiek, H.F., Randell, R., Breeden, J.A., Chambers, J.E. and Murphy, J.R. (1966). The thermal conductivity measurements and predictions for biological fluids and tissues. Cryobiology, **3**, 318-27
12. Lipkin, M. and Hardy, J.D. (1954). Measurement of some thermal properties of human tissues. J. Appl. Physiol., **7**, 212-17
13. Stoll, A.M. and Greene, L.C. (1959). Relationship between pain and tissue damage due to thermal radiation. J. Appl. Physiol., **14**, 373-87
14. Hensel, H. and Bender, F. (1956). Fortlanfende Bestimmang der Hautdurchblutung am Menschen mit einem elekrtischen Warmeleitmesser. Pfluegers Arch. Ges. Physiol., **263**, 603-14
15. Brown, B.H., Bygrave, C., Robinson, P. and Henderson, H.P. (1980). A critique of the use of a thermal clearance probe for the measurement of skin blood flow. Clin. Phys. Physiol. Meas., **1**, 237-41
16. Pennes, H.H. (1948). Analysis of tissue and arterial blood temperatures in the resting human forearm. J. Appl. Physiol., **1**, 93-122
17. Carslaw, H.S. and Jaeger, J.C. (1959). Conduction of Heat in Solids. 2nd edn. (Oxford: Oxford University Press)
18. Patterson, A.M. (1976). Transient heat transfer in the superficial tissues of the forearm after a step-change in surrounding air temperature. Research Report No.71, University of the Witwatersrand, RSA, School of Mechanical Engineering
19. Hodson, D.A., Eason, G. and Barbenel, J.C. (1986). Modelling transient heat transfer through the skin and superficial tissues: 1. Surface insulation. J. Biomed. Eng., **106**, 183-8

Chapter 21

The acoustic properties of the epidermis and stratum corneum

C Edwards

INTRODUCTION

When ultrasound is used to measure or image skin or its components, the information obtained relates only to the variations of the acoustic impedance of the object. Radiography displays a map of electron density of tissue, and electron microscopy gives topological information on the electron density of prepared tissue sections. The familiar light microscope reveals only tissue structures which take up the stains used and transmit light of certain wavelengths. Even then its apparent structure can vary enormously with specimen preparation. In contrast, ultrasound is used to interrogate the skin to reveal its mechanical structure.

One large difference between ultrasound and other methods seems to be that, while the dependence of the perceived image on imaging method is accepted and used in a positive way with other methods, the anatomical origin of the ultrasound image or data is less clearly understood. At the very least, no publication has produced a reasoned explanation of echogenicity in skin and associated tissues. The most obvious comparison of ultrasound skin thickness measurement with other methods has, to date, simply shown X-ray pictures against A-scan echograms with no justification for the A-scan interpretation[1]. After the interpretation of the anatomical correspondence to the received echo data has been resolved (or taken for granted), the next step is the measurement of the data. In the simplest case of the A-scan thickness measurement, then the time between echoes from two structures within the skin is measured and multiplied by the velocity of sound in the tissue to arrive at the thickness measurement. The velocity chosen will of course determine the 'measured' thickness. Some justification or measurement of this velocity is required. So an acoustic description of skin should supply, or at least indicate, two pieces of information: firstly, an idea of what components of skin are likely to produce echo data so that clear confident interpretation of skin A-scans and B-scans is possible; secondly, a figure for the velocity of sound in the various skin layers would enable accurate dimensional information to be gained from echo data.

In this chapter it is proposed to concentrate on the stratum corneum and underlying epidermis, which are of great interest to dermatologists, pharmacologists and cosmetic scientists.

STRATUM CORNEUM

The stratum corneum presents the first layer of skin to an acoustic beam. This layer will vary in composition, thickness and surface roughness at various body sites[2]. For hairy non-friction no-load bearing skin the stratum corneum consists of 8-15 cell layers each somewhat less than 1 μm thick: the cells are polygonal and measure some 40 μm in their longest dimensions. The top layers of cells are in equilibrium with the outside environment, which leads to water content as low as 5 mg water per 100 mg dry weight, but with a typical content of higher than 20 mg water per 100 mg dry weight. This compares with a figure of about 400 mg water per 100 mg dry weight for most internal tissues. So, for the purpose of acoustic propagation, the stratum corneum can almost be considered as a solid. However, the upper layers of this tissue are highly hydrophilic and when immersed in water swell considerably[2]. This hydration will have a profound effect on the velocity, C, density, D, and hence specific acoustic impedance, Z ($Z = CD$) of the horny layer. The usual acoustic coupling medium used in A-scan is water or water-based gel. Consequently the transit time of a pulse through the stratum corneum will alter because first the layer will swell as it takes up water; and second, the velocity of sound will change as the composition alters from the initial dry state to the fully hydrated state when immersed.

Thus for thickness measurement of stratum corneum it is essential to use a non-aqueous medium such as mineral oil, or to occlude the skin surface with a water repellant, or to attempt to correct for the swelling effect of the water coupling medium. This is relatively unimportant when measuring non-load bearing whole skin, in which the stratum corneum thickness (about 10-20 μm)[3] is such a small part of total dermal thickness (1-3 mm), but would be important on measurement of palmar or plantar skin, where the stratum corneum can by typically 600 μm thick[2], or in skin with an abnormally thickened epidermis.

Histologically, there is a sharp distinction between stratum granulosum and stratum corneum. The cells of the granular layer are living and filled with cytoplasm. The horny layer cells are dead and completely keratinized. However, the amount of keratin in the cells does not change as abruptly as the morphology would suggest but shows a more gradual maturation from keratin precursors in the prickle cell layer. Only in the stratum corneum is the keratin stable or 'mature' and contributes to the hard outer horny layer. The velocity and density changes between stratum corneum and stratum granulosum would therefore arise mainly from different degrees of hydration - there being less water in the dead stratum corneum than in the living stratum granulosum.

The cells of the stratum corneum are more tightly packed than elsewhere in the epidermis and so present a more solid layer of hardened protein than any other layer. Therefore, it would be expected that the attenuation of ultrasound would be greatest within this layer. Certainly, in the hard friction pads of palmar and plantar epidermis the stratified squamous layers would cause scattering and possibly structural resonance absorption giving high attenuation. In the loosely constructed parakeratotic stratum corneum seen in certain skin disorders the poor contact seen between strata would cause greater attenuation than in normal skin.

The surface roughness of the stratum corneum is also a factor to be considered. In normal skin the rete ridge depth may approach the stratum corneum depth giving rise to an ill-defined upper surface. The lower surface is over most of the body relatively smooth allowing for a clear acoustic boundary to be established if the stratum corneum is not too water-logged.

The following points summarize the acoustic properties of stratum corneum:

(1) The stratum corneum is distinguishable as a separate clearly defined layer by the change in water content from the stratum granulosum. Therefore acoustic contrast is lessened when the skin is immersed in water and it is best to use a non-penetrating non-aqueous coupling medium if stratum corneum thickness is required.

(2) The stratum corneum should exhibit higher attenuation than the other skin layers because of its dry stratified structure.

(3) The lower surface should appear flat and give a clear echo. The upper surface will appear rough to an acoustic pulse of sufficient bandwidth to measure its thickness (except on load-bearing stratum corneum). Therefore it is probably best to use an unfocused beam to measure stratum corneum thickness which will average out surface features and indicate a 'mean' surface.

(4) The velocity of sound in the stratum corneum is likely to be higher than in other layers because of the presence of hard keratin.

(5) The acoustic impedance and hence the reflectivity of this layer will depend markedly on its state of hydration. For lowest impedance and thus the best coupling of sound through the stratum corneum it should be highly hydrated or water-logged.

EPIDERMIS

The epidermis is seldom more than about 70 μm thick, except on load-bearing surfaces, and ranges from about 15 to 50 μm on the abdomen, thorax and limbs. The acoustic properties of the epidermis will depend on the inclusions present in any particular area as well as the generally constant propagation properties of the cellular structure. In particular, there will be a striking difference between glabrous and hairy epidermis. The water content of these layers is about 60-80%, in common with most body tissues, and the velocity in the cellular matrix would be about the same as in other mainly cellular tissues[4], about 1540 m s^{-1}. The inclusion of hair shafts and glandular tubules will have a small effect on the overall velocity through the layer, the magnitude and sign of which it is difficult to predict. Certainly, scalp epidermis should show a different velocity from palmar or plantar epidermis.

The upper boundary of the stratum malpighii, the stratum granulosum is relatively flat and the reflection behaviour is that discussed in considering stratum corneum. The lower margin is clearly marked histologically by the thin basement membrane on which grows the basal cell layer. This membrane separates the continuous closely packed cellular basal layer from the loose collagenous vascularized dermis, and should therefore represent a significant acoustic impedance change. Clearly, here the acoustic image will exactly conform to the histological structure. Unfortunately, the dermo-epidermal junction is by no means flat. Not only do the epidermal appendages penetrate into the dermis, but also the dermal papillae project into the epidermis causing numerous pits to be formed in its under surface. These papillae contain capillary loops from which the epidermis obtains its nutrients, so in areas of high epidermal activity such as friction surfaces and hair growing areas such as scalp, the papillae will be more numerous. So the dermo-epidermal junction will give a strong echo exactly following the anatomical junction, which means that a flat transducer will give the best results for a mean epidermal depth. A focused beam may be deflected by the epidermal appendages and by the sides of the dermal papillae. However, a good echo can be obtained from the peaks and troughs alike, allowing a measurement of maximum and minimum epidermal thickness. Glabrous skin will give the least complicated signal because of the lack of hair shaft inclusions.

The attenuation in the epidermis should be much the same as for the other body cellular tissues. The absorption will be as for normal tissues, mainly because the cells are in contact via lymph, and no gross structures except hair shafts would cause relaxational absorption.

Scattering will occur mainly from hair shafts since hair keratin has such a different acoustic impedance compared to cellular tissue (being much harder, with consequent increase in elastic modulus) and these structures are probably the only ones which would give significant echoes (that is, echoes which may confuse the dermo-epidermal junction echo). In hairy areas such as scalp, the scattering from hair shafts may increase the attenuation of the beam.

The acoustic properties of the epidermis can be summarised as follows:

(1) The epidermis is distinguishable as an acoustic layer by a very well defined acoustic boundary at the basement membrane, and an upper stratum corneum boundary dependent on the water content of stratum corneum. The lower surface is not flat: its

mean position may be obtained from a flat transducer, and its maximum and minimum positions from a finely focused beam.

(2) It will have an attenuation roughly the same as other soft tissues, except in very hairy areas where scattering may remove energy from the beam. This effect will vary with frequency and beam width. To minimize this effect a low-frequency wide beam should be used, which may be acceptable on scalp areas since its thickness allows a lower bandwidth signal to be used.

(3) The velocity of sound in epidermis should be much the same as for other soft tissues, i.e. about 1540 m s^{-1}.

(4) The acoustic impedance of epidermis should be about the same as for soft tissues, which allows this layer to be distinguished from the stratum corneum and the dermis, both of which exhibit markedly different impedances.

MEASURED PROPERTIES

There are sparse data in the literature on the acoustic properties of human skin, and almost no data on properties of its component layers. The major problem with the published data is that without exception not enough experimental details are published to allow comparisons between workers, or even to know exactly from what tissue or from what species measurements were made.

Table 21.1 Previously published values for acoustic velocity in skin

Author	Value (m s^{-1})	Comments
Dussik et al.[5]	1498	Unspecified 'skin' in vitro
Daly and Wheeler[6]	1518	Unspecified 'skin' in vitro
Goans et al.[7]	1540	Limited number of experiments on human eschar
Edwards[8]	1580	Deduced from acoustic considerations of skin composition

Table 21.1 illustrates this with the previously published values for acoustic velocity in whole skin - no published figures are yet available for isolated stratum corneum or epidermis. Also, data are not available from in vivo experiments, since independent accurate measurements of individual skin layer thicknesses are extremely difficult to obtain.

The only data available for attenuation (expressed as a loss of signal strength in decibels per unit thickness in centimetres) is for whole skin and subcutaneous fat, published in 1958[5]. This is presented in Table 21.2. However, these measurements were made a.

three single, continuous low frequencies and low power levels. This means that it is impossible to extrapolate from these results any realistic estimate of attenuation values expected using the short high intensity pulses (containing a range of frequencies typically from 10 MHz to 30 MHz) used in the present day A-scan examination of skin structure.

Table 21.2 Previously published values for acoustic propagation constants of skin

Author	Values	Comments
Dussik et al.[5]	α = 3.5 (dB cm^{-1}) 7.4 9.2	1 MHz Unspecified 'skin' 3 MHz 5 MHz
Dussik et al.[5]	α = 0.6 (dB cm^{-1}) 1.6 2.3	1 MHz Unspecified adipose tissue 3 MHz 5 MHz
Ogura et al.[9]	Z = 1.5-1.7 Rayls	In vivo, 37°C, from a range of sites
Edwards[8]	Z = 1.534 Rayls Z = 1.519 Rayls	Palmar stratum corneum Epidermis

Table 21.2 presents results from the only two reports of measurements of the acoustic impedance of skin. This is analogous to the refractive index of substances for light propagation and determines the reflectivity and hence the 'acoustic contrast' of tissues. As stated previously, the acoustic impedance, Z, is directly related to the density, D, of tissue (Z = C x D), but it is also related to the elastic modulus, E by Z = $\sqrt{}$(D x E). This relationship is used to directly and non-invasively measure absolute values and changes in values of elastic properties of materials in many areas of engineering, and should also be of value in tissue characterization measurements.

Table 21.3 presents data which enables the fundamental equations quoted above to be used to estimate the speed of sound in and the acoustic impedance of skin tissue from independent measurements of the density[10] and the bulk elastic modulus[11], using stratum corneum as an example. The derived results for Z from Table 21.3 are in remarkable agreement with the measured values reported in Table 21.2[8,9].

Table 21.3 Stratum corneum acoustic properties derived from published data

Average density, D (ref.10)	1.1×10^3 kg m^{-3}
Elastic modulus, E (ref.11)*	2×10^9 N m^{-2}
Sound velocity, C (C = $\sqrt{}$(E/D)	1.35×10^3 m s^{-1}
Acoustic impedance, Z (Z = D x C)	1.48 Rayls

N.B. 1 Rayl = 1×10^6 kg m^{-2} s^{-1}
* Elastic modulus figure quoted for 30% relative humidity

Table 21.4 Acoustic constants in skin measured in a recent study

	Density $(kg\ m^{-3} \times 10^{-3})$	Velocity $(m\ s^{-1})$	Impedance (Rayls)
Whole skin	1.1764	1583	1.863
Epidermis	1.106	1500	1.659
Dermis	1.274	1660	2.115

Table 21.4 shows preliminary results from in vitro measurements of propagation constants made in Cardiff. The densities were measured using the Percol density bead marked density gradient method[12]. The velocity was obtained from whole and heat-separated skin by independent measurement of sample thickness and acoustic pulse transit time.

CONCLUSION

The work of establishing accurate ranges for acoustic propagation constants in human skin is essential if A-scan and B-scan ultrasound are to aid dermatological diagnosis or are to provide tools for assessment of the physical changes occurring during therapy. This work has begun in Cardiff and results confirm the theoretical estimates. In the future it is hoped that such data will enable the use of ultrasound as a non-invasive method for dermatological tissue characterization.

REFERENCES

1. Alexander, H. and Miller, D. (1979). Determining skin thickness with pulsed ultrasound. J. Invest. Dermatol., 72, 17-19
2. Kligman, A.M. (1964). The biology of the stratum corneum. In Montagna, W. and Lobitz, W.C. (eds.) The Epidermis. (New York: Academic Press)
3. Holbrook, K.A. and Odland, G.F. (1974). Regional differences in the thickness (cell layers) of the human stratum corneum: an ultrastructural analysis. J. Invest. Dermatol., 62, 415-22
4. Chivers, R.C. and Parry, R.J. (1978). Ultrasonic velocity and attenuation in mammalian tissues. J. Acoustical Soc. Am., 63(3), 940-53
5. Dussik, K.T., Fritch, D.J., Kyriazidou, M. and Sears, R.S. (1958). Measurements of articular tissues with ultrasound. Am. J. Phys. Med., 37, 160-5
6. Daly, C.H. and Wheeler, J.B. (1971). The use of ultrasonic thickness measurement in clinical measurement of the oral soft tissue. Int. Dent. J., 21(4), 418-29
7. Goans, R.E., Cantrell, J.H. and Myers, F.B. (1977). Ultrasonic pulse-echo determination of thermal injury in deep dermal burns. Med. Phys., 4, 259-63
8. Edwards, C. (1984). The use of high frequency ultrasound to study dimensions and properties of skin. PhD Thesis, University of Manchester Faculty of Technology
9. Ogura, I., Kidokoro, T., Iinuma, K., Tanaka, K. and Matsuda, A. (1978). Measurement of acoustic impedance of skin. In White, D.N. and Lyons, E.A. (eds.) Ultrasound in Medicine, Vol.4. (New York: Plenum Press)
10. Weigand, D.A., Haygood, C. and Gaylor, J.R. (1974). Cell layers and density of Negro and Caucasian stratum corneum. J. Invest. Dermatol., 62, 563-8
11. Park, A.C. and Baddiel, C.B. (1972). Rheology of stratum corneum.2. A physicochemical investigation of factors influencing the water content of the corneum. J. Soc. Cosmetic Chem., 23, 13-21
12. Thomas, S.E., Dykes, P.J. and Marks, R. (1985). Plantar hyperkeratosis: a study of callosities and normal plantar skin. J. Invest. Dermatol., 85, 394-7

Chapter 22

The electrical properties of skin

C Edwards

INTRODUCTION

The skin exhibits extremely complex electrical properties, which, although related to its physical and chemical state, are not readily amenable to interpretation in these terms. In order to extract useful information from measurement of skin electrical properties, a means of relating the physical state of the skin to its observed electrical behaviour is required. Thus a model or models needs to be proposed to allow the design of measurement methods.

One common model involves the construction of 'equivalent circuits' where certain skin components are assumed to behave like electrical devices, put together in various combinations or circuits[1]. Then standard electrical theory predicts the behaviour of such circuits in various measurement configurations. The main disadvantage of this method is that the true electrical behaviour of skin is so complex that no equivalent circuit can be constructed which holds true for anything more than a single, often unrealistic, set of physical constraints on the measurement conditions. The other approach attempts to model the skin in terms of the theories of solid state physics[2]. Although initially daunting in complexity, this latter approach may prove the more rewarding.

For either approach it must be stated that factors such as site, mechanical deformation, temperature, relative humidity, injury, pathological conditions, surface materials, nervous state of the subjects and instrumental variables are all well known to affect the precise values of the components of the mathematical equations which are consequently almost impossible to predict[3].

CONSIDERATIONS FOR MEASUREMENT TECHNIQUES

The main reasons for trying to use measurements of electrical properties to assess skin are that;

(1) The method is non-invasive,

(2) The relative change in electrical properties with change in skin structure or function is larger than with other physical changes, i.e. the method is potentially very sensitive,

(3) Since the measurements are mainly confined to the surface layer of skin[4] the method is 'tuned' for stratum corneum.

For adequate characterization of the electrical properties of skin, its electrical behaviour must be measured over as wide a range of frequencies as possible. This entails measuring both real and imaginary components of the impedance presented by the skin[5]. This can be difficult and, since it requires complex instrumentation, expensive[6]. For optimum reproducibility, accuracy and reduction of systematic errors, as many as possible of the ambient and internal variables which affect the skin's electrical behaviour must be controlled. Also of supreme importance is the electrical coupling of the skin to the instrumentation, the electrodes. Their configuration (shape, area, material), number, site, distribution and coupling method must be standardized and repeatable.

Once a set of data has been obtained, it must be fitted to an appropriate model, and coefficients determined. Then the model will transform the electrical measurement set into physical or chemical skin properties. In order that the method is accepted as adequate for its purpose, some independent verification of its results is required, i.e. it has to be 'calibrated' or tested against a set of known values of the skin properties of interest.

ELECTRICAL PROPERTIES

The main electrical properties of stratum corneum which form the basis of the semiconductor model of skin behaviour are given below. These statements are generally true for normal skin, but may not hold in abnormal stratum corneum or when topical agents have been applied whose electrical behaviour may 'swamp' that of the skin.

The characteristic curves of applied current versus observed voltage are non-linear. This behaviour is due to the presence of the fixed charge on the proteins of the stratum corneum[7]. Thus it can clearly be stated that skin is non-ohmic in its electrical behaviour.

The direct current conductance of non-dry powdered keratin (not stratum corneum) is thermally activated, behaving like an intrinsic semiconductor[8]. The conductors are probably protonic, but changes in conduction lag behind hydration changes. This effect is caused by the fact that water in the stratum corneum is bound in three states - strongly bound, weakly bound and free (see Chapter 17) - so conduction through the stratum corneum is not linearly related to the water content. In general, as the water content within the stratum corneum increases, the amount bound and the binding strength decrease, increasing the permittivity. This increase in permittivity is caused by the plasticizing of polypeptide side-chains of keratin, allowing easier charge transfer between molecules. This also decreases the semiconductor activation energy.

SEMICONDUCTOR THEORY OF SKIN ELECTRICAL PROPERTIES

Using the above information, a theory which predicts skin electrical behaviour can be proposed[2] if the following additional assumptions are made:

(1) That the conduction process can be modelled by charge transfer in a random system,

(2) That identical charge trapping sites exist, separated by random distances, and

(3) That Coulombic interactions generate a distribution of potential barriers between trap sites.

In descriptive terms it can be supposed that the proteins in skin exhibit small energy gaps between their conduction and valence bands. A few electrons can be excited to energy levels between the two bands where they remain for a short time during which charge may be carried (extrinsic semiconduction). These intermediate energy levels are called localized states, and the mean residency time for a particular electron is the relaxation time. The effect of these relaxation times is to produce an effective capacitance, such as is found in transistors. It is this capacitance that gives the imaginary (non-DC, frequency dependent) conduction.

The theory, and supporting experimental evidence, show that for a particular amplitude of sinusoidal stimulation, the alternating current complex electrical impedance, Z, of skin has the following form:

$$Z(\omega) = R_\infty + \frac{R_0 - R_\infty}{1 + (j\omega\tau_p)^{1-m}} \qquad (1)$$

where:

ω = 2π times the sinusoidal excitation frequency,
R_∞ = series resistance at high values of ω ($\omega\tau_p \gg 1$),
R_0 = series resistance at very low frequencies,
τ_p = mean relaxation time.

m is related to width of distribution curve of relaxation times, and takes values between 0 and 1.

This is equivalent to the Cole equation[9]. This equation can be rewritten in the form:

$$Z(\omega) = R_s(\omega) + jX_s(\omega) \qquad (2)$$

where $R_s(\omega)$ is the (real) series resistance, and $X_s(\omega)$ is the (imaginary) series reactance. It is in this form that impedance measurements are made, and the output graph of $X_s(\omega)$ vs. $R_s(\omega)$ takes the form shown in Figure 22.1.

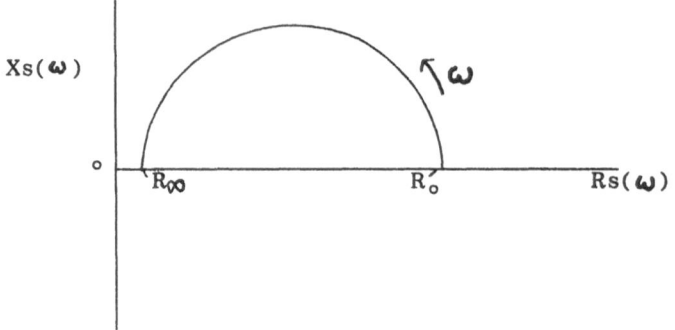

Figure 22.1 Plot of $R_s(\omega)$ vs. $X_s(\omega)$, i.e. locus of $Z(\omega)$

The theory proposed by Salter[2] predicts equation 1 exactly, and proposes reasonable interpretations for its constituent factors. For example, the number m in equation 1 is found to be given as

$$m = \frac{4kT}{S - SX}$$

where:

K = Boltzmann's constant,
T = temperature (absolute),
S = trap energy at infinite separation,
$X = \dfrac{KT}{S} (\log_e[1/\omega\tau])$,
ω = 2π times excitation frequency,
τ = relaxation time constant.

For reasonable parameter values, this equation does give m values between 0 and 1, in accord with the Cole equation. It also shows that m is (1) dependent on temperature, (2) only weakly dependent on frequency, and (3) dependent on electrical trap energies, S. Observation (3) means that m is dependent on the intrinsic properties of the stratum corneum proteins, and may therefore be used as a measurand.

MEASUREMENTS ON SKIN

The use of single frequency measurements of skin conductance is fraught with difficulties, since such measurements are not unique descriptors of skin properties. Also the effects of sweating, emotional state, contact resistance and nerve impulse fields are difficult to assess. Another major difficulty is that the effects of hydration, temperature and skin structures are not separable at one

212

frequency. However, for relative measurements, where changes occurring after modulation of one factor (e.g. skin hydration with emollient cream) are monitored, the single frequency method may be adequate.

The use of a full frequency-dependent electrical impedance measurement will yield more reliable and reproducible results which have the support of a reasonable theory behind their interpretation in terms of stratum corneum properties. However, the investment in terms of equipment, expertise, experimental control and data analysis is great, and may deter many from this method.

Although measurements of skin electrical properties have been proposed for characterizing the effects of pathological change[5,10], the results are usually too variable to be of any direct clinical use. By far the most widespread use of the technique is for assessment of the effects of drugs and cosmetics. More specifically, the method is used to detect the 'moisturizing' effects of emollients. For this purpose, simple single-frequency measurements may suffice, providing that the applied substance does not contain, for example, penetrating resistive oils, which in themselves alter the stratum corneum resistivity independently of the increased water-retaining capacity under investigation[11].

For a more reliable and thorough measurement of moisturization separated from the effects of other components, a multifrequency method must be used[12]. This entails much more complex instrumentation and data analysis, but the results of changes due to treatment are clearly displayed.

REFERENCES

1. Edelberg, R. (1971). Electrical properties of skin. In Elden, H.R. (ed.) Biophysical Properties of the Skin. pp 513-50. (New York: Wiley, Interscience)
2. Salter, D.C. (1981). Studies in the measurement, form and interpretation of some electrical properties of normal and pathological skin in vivo. DPhil Thesis, University of Oxford, England
3. Millington, P.F. and Wilkinson, R. (1983). Skin. In Harrison, R.J. and McMinn, R.M.H. (eds.) Biological Structure and Function. Vol. 9, pp 127-42. (Cambridge, England: Cambridge University Press)
4. Yamamoto, T. and Yamamoto, Y. (1976). Electrical properties of the epidermal stratum corneum. Med. Biol. Eng. Comput., 14, 151
5. Yamamoto, T. and Yamamoto, Y. (1977). Analysis for the change in skin impedance. Med. Biol. Eng. Comput., 15, 219
6. Salter, D.C. (1981). Alternating current electrical properties of human skin measured in vivo. In Marks, R. and Payne, P. (eds.) Bioengineering and the Skin. p 267. (Lancaster, England: MTP Press)
7. Rosendal, T. (1943). Studies on the conducting properties of human skin to direct and alternating current. Acta Physiol. Scand., 5, 130
8. Pethig, R. (1979). Dielectric and Electronic Properties of Biological Materials. (Chichester, England: John Wiley & Sons)
9. Cole, K.S. (1940). Permeability and impermeability of cell membranes for ions. Cold Spring Harbour Symposium. Quantitative Biol., 4, 10
10. Woodrough, R.E., Cauti, G. and Watson, B.W. (1975). Electrical potential difference between basal cell carcinoma, benign inflammatory lesions and normal tissue. Br. J. Dermatol., 92, 1-7
11. Clar, E.J., Her, C.P. and Sturelle, C.G. (1975). Skin impedance and moisturization. J. Soc. Cosmet. Chem., 26, 337-53
12. Yamamoto, Y., Yamamoto, T., Ohta, S., Uehara, T., Tahara, S. and Ishizuka, Y. (1978). The measurement principle for evaluating the performance of drugs and cosmetics by skin impedance. Med. Biol. Eng. Comput., 16, 623-32

Index